Carla Oates is the founder and CEO of The Beauty Chef – a brand that launched the global inner beauty market. Since the creation of her first product GLOW® Inner Beauty Essential in 2009, Carla has continued to pioneer the global ingestible beauty category, educating her community on the power of the gut-skin connection and the importance of the gut microbiome for health, beauty and wellbeing.

Carla lives in Bondi with her husband, her two adult children (sometimes) and her dog Wolfie. When she isn't working on new products, she loves spending time in the garden or the kitchen – combining the joy of cooking with the science of nutrition.

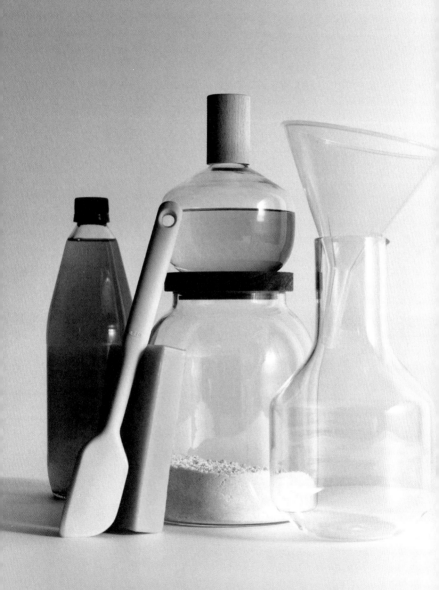

Feeding Your Skin

CARLA OATES

Hardie Grant

BOOKS

*For Jeet and Otis, husband Davor and to my beautiful late mum,
for her unconditional love and support, always.*

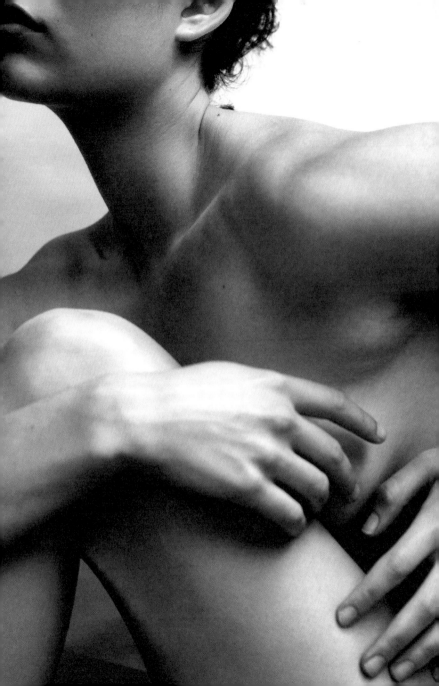

Contents

Preface

When I first wrote this book more than two decades ago, the idea of 100% natural, organic and clean beauty products was quite a foreign concept. But since then, there has been an incredible shift in the beauty space and it's been wonderful to witness the progress made, as well as the emergence of new brands where the makers have been conscious of the ingredients they use and the impact they have on our health and the environment.

Although much has changed for the better – and I have since launched my own brand that speaks to the importance of gut health not only for skin health, but also our overall vitality and wellbeing – a lot of what I wrote in this book still rings true today. This is why the re-release of *Feeding Your Skin* excites me just as much as it did when I spent weekends crafting and curating each recipe the first time around.

Now, with a slight modern makeover, *Feeding Your Skin* is an even more gorgeous guide to creating nutritious, homemade recipes that will nuture your skin's microbiome, support its natural barrier and leave you feeling utterly radiant. For anyone looking to take care of their skin by preparing their own fresh, toxin-free formulations, this book will be a precious resource.

But first, let's go back to the beginning ...

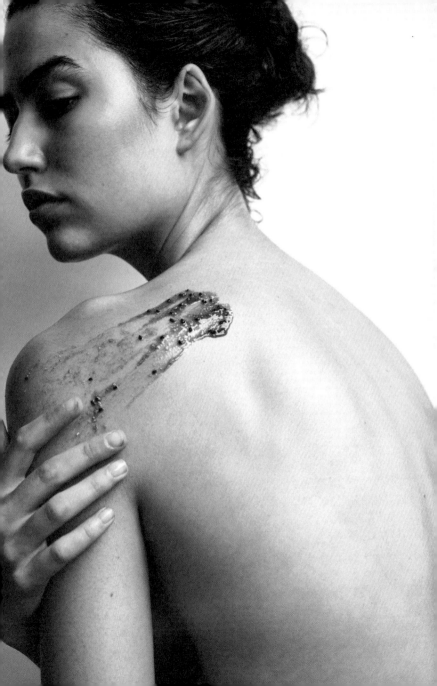

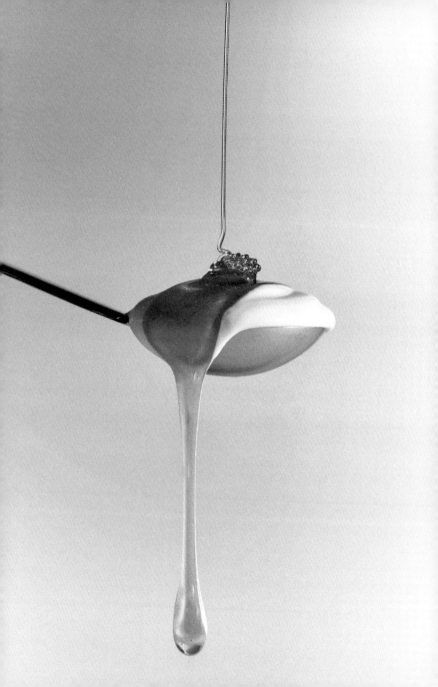

Introduction

As small children, my sister and I delighted in concocting wild and wonderful lotions and potions. My mum called us the 'little witches' as we spent hours upon days furtively mixing together her perfumes and cosmetics with all sorts of odds and ends from the kitchen cupboard and clippings from the garden. Before long, I had set up a healing clinic in the lounge room and employed our finest brews to help cure the imaginary skin conditions of any willing and brave patient (namely our parents). For my 'magic', we charged a small fortune.

So, as fate (and a few decades later) would have it, I found myself a beauty editor, both surrounded by and prescribing readers all sorts of ointments, creams, balms, treatments and makeup on the market. Only sadly, as I came to discover, the ones in the fancy packaging contained very little magic at all. In our quest to look good, we had indiscriminately forsaken the knowledge handed down by generations – that of nutritious homemade cosmetic recipes. Long before we started looking to the shelves for solutions, skin was taken care of using fresh wholesome ingredients, whipped up centuries before mainstream companies began promising perfect skin and luscious hair.

When exploring the ingredient lists of products during those years, the most favoured cosmetics were made with chemical solvents and synthetic additives – questionable substances that may over time be absorbed into the body through the skin and compromise our wellbeing. Even the pots of goo that were trading under the 'green' banner were often full of undesirable ingredients.

Life as a beauty editor put me high up in the popularity stakes – I was sent loads of products – and at times I felt like the local beauty pusher. My house became the preferred venue for family lunches. The meal was usually followed by a casual utterance, 'Oh, by the way, I need a new moisturiser'. Invariably we'd end up in what my daughter called 'mummy's product room'. That was until I started driving the 'go natural' bandwagon and placed an indefinite embargo on the (questionable) product room. Instead, I 'progressed' back to childhood, concocting my own special toxin-free formulations for the skin and bottling them. I'd stick pretty pictures on the bottles to seduce my otherwise dubious friends, offering them as substitutes for mainstream brands. By the time I had developed my first inner beauty product for The Beauty Chef, GLOW® years later, my friends were more than used to receiving DIY-beauty products courtesy of my kitchen!

To complement my packaged goods, I'd also create delicious and nutritious fresh-food facials, crack eggs into the hair, slather avocado onto the skin, apply sugar scrubs to the body and wax legs with sticky, buttery toffee. A wonderful rich, nutritious and tactile feast for the skin and hair, created using fresh and organic ingredients found in the fridge and bowl – without one harmful ingredient. The responses from my guinea pigs were very positive. Radiant skin and fun-filled afternoon cosmetic cook-ups inspired comments like 'You should open a salon' or 'Write a book that I can keep alongside my favourite recipe books in the kitchen.' A cookbook for the skin? Brilliant!

This book is full of creative and delicious recipes and ideas to give you back the power of caring for your body. It is dedicated to anyone who wants to nurture their skin and body kindly and safely. Over the years, it has become very apparent to me that those who anoint themselves with the purest of oils and botanical concoctions have the most radiant, dewy skin. This is enhanced by their holistic approach to beauty; they eat well, exercise and engage in activities that give them joy. After all, joy truly is the best cosmetic! The other advantage of looking after yourself holistically is that you are contributing to a happier and healthier environment – only pure, unadulterated ingredients will be washed into our precious seas.

The recipes in this book come from myriad sources. For some recipes, I was inspired by kitchen alchemists who have gone before me and by the time-honoured remedies from ancient cultures, including the wonderful world of Ayurvedic beauty. Others recipes have come from the inspiring people I have met on my journey – my beautiful mum, who was the first person to show me how powerful a natural approach to health and wellbeing could be, as well as natural health practitioners who have dedicated themselves to educating individuals on how to empower themselves. The rest come from me, after the hours I have spent experimenting in my kitchen – a creative adventure of sorts that has not only altered the way I look after my skin, but also inspired my journey to create The Beauty Chef years later.

INNER BEAUTY

While the recipes in this book will promote healthy and radiant skin, remember that topical treatments work best alongside a diet rich in antioxidants, enzymes and other proteins, vitamins, essential fatty acids, minerals, prebiotics and probiotics. I am forever telling my friends who complain about their skin to spend their money on a naturopath rather than a beautician – and to continue nourishing their gut, first and foremost. The skin, hair and nails are the last stop for essential nutrients (which go to the most important organs first), so it's of the utmost importance to maintain a balanced diet and support a thriving gut microbiome and to consult with a naturopath to ensure you are assimilating nutrients properly. They will also work with you to ensure your body is eliminating toxins efficiently through the liver and kidneys, so all the impurities don't flood through your skin and cause skin conditions. Premature ageing of the skin can also be related to sun damage, stress, hormonal changes, pollution, lack of exercise, and too much sugar and refined foods – so it's not just about what we put on our face.

Confidence and contentment give your face a radiance that cannot be replicated by makeup, as disturbances in the skin may reflect an emotional world out of balance. This is why it's so important to nuture your mental wellbeing – speak to a therapist, move mindfully, practise meditation and always endeavour to surround yourself with positive people who make you feel accepted and loved. Reducing your stress levels in this way will inevitably improve your complexion – even without any special treatments. So take a deep breath, drink lots of clean, filtered water, feed your skin and find the joy in the every day.

SKIN TYPES

There are generally accepted skin types. This classification is based on the balance of water and sebum in the tissues.

NORMAL is rare unless you're very young. It is soft, smooth, finely textured, supple and balanced in both oil and moisture content. It has no enlarged pores, wrinkles or blemishes and is firm and resilient.

OILY has a coarser texture, with obvious enlarged pores. The skin may look sallow or shiny and is prone to acne, blackheads and infection. It's greasy as a result of overproduction of sebum, which can be caused by a number of factors, including genetics, bad diet, metabolic disorders, hormonal imbalances, insufficient skin hygiene or harsh preparations that strip the oil from the skin.

DRY is usually delicate and fine-textured, with no obvious pores, and has a predisposition to facial lines and wrinkles. It lacks moisture or fat due to inadequate production by the sebaceous glands and an inability to trap surface moisture. Often it feels tight, parched and flaky.

COMBINATION is a mixture of two or more skin types. Often, this looks like dry patches with oily patches on the T-zones, where the sebaceous glands are most prevalent: the forehead, nose and chin. Each area is best treated according to its needs. For example, two types of mask should be prepared, one for each skin type.

SENSITIVE is fine-textured and translucent, and often prone to lines and small surface veins. It can suffer redness and irritation when exposed to allergens in the air and to products such as perfume, lanolin and pollen. It is often more susceptible to eczema and dermatitis. People with this skin type are often very sensitive and finely tuned both physically and emotionally.

Skin concerns

DEHYDRATED is lacking in water, quickly wrinkled, drawn and often cold. Lack of water in the tissues can be caused by insufficient fluid intake, poor lymphatic function, dieting, climatic conditions, spending time in heated or air-conditioned spaces, or lack of sebum. Both dry and oily skin types can become dehydrated.

MATURE OR AGEING is prone to dryness and dehydration, as it lacks oil and moisture, and to wrinkles and lines. The skin can feel loose or sag (due to underlying fat-shrinkage and a loss of collagen), or appear dull. Growths and pigmentation occur, and small capillaries appear.

ACNEOUS suffers from acne, a skin condition, which has myriad underlying causes, but is often due to an overproduction of sebum and blocked hair follicles. This excess sebum can lead to blackheads, skin inflammation and pimples.

BROKEN CAPILLARIES appear as small, dilated, winding, bright red blood vessels on the cheeks, around the nose and sometimes on the chin. Broken capillaries occur as a result of poor elasticity of the capillary wall and they give the appearance of diffuse or local redness. Broken capillaries are aggravated by extremes of temperature, by swimming or bathing in excessively hot or cold water, nervous or digestive disorders, poor nutrition, spending time in saunas, exercise, drinking very hot liquids, eating spicy foods, blushing, smoking, drinking alcohol, and using aggressive scrubs and alcohol-based toners.

Where
to begin

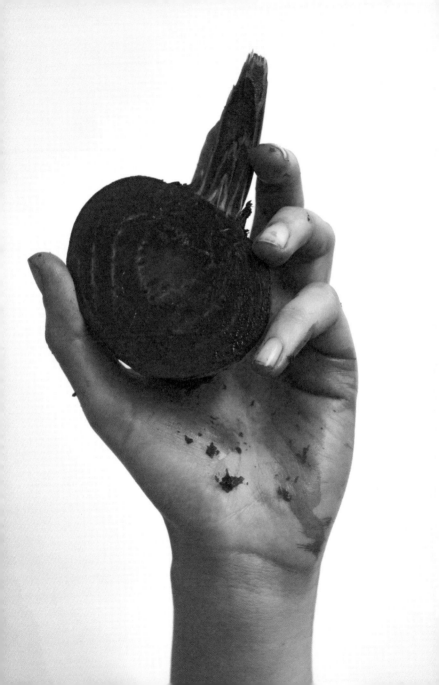

The essential ingredients

You don't need a masters in chemistry to create nourishing skincare when the latest buzz ingredients are found in the most humble of foods. Fruits, flowers, veggies, herbs, dairy products, beans, nuts and flours are rich in essential vitamins, minerals, fruit acids, enzymes, amino acids, alpha-hydroxy acids (AHAs), fatty acids, antioxidants, carbohydrates, proteins, pre, pro and postbiotics – which are all the active ingredients you need to create luxurious and sophisticated skincare.

Creating your own skincare may be a little time consuming, but if you dedicate a day every so often to replenishing your supplies, it can evolve into a nurturing beauty ritual, inspiring you to take time out and care for your body and skin in a truly holistic way. Gather a group of friends and make a day of cosmetic cooking. That way you can share the costs and time, and swap your delicious recipes.

There's no pressure to replace all the products in your routine with DIY options; mark your favourites to come back to and use alongside clean, quality products from brands you trust. The recipes in this book are easy and many of them cost very little, putting handcrafted beauty and wellbeing within anyone's reach.

THE SKIN'S SAVIOURS

ANTIOXIDANTS fight free radicals. Vibrantly coloured fruits, veggies and herbs are rich in carotenoids, such as lutein, beta-carotene, lycopene and alpha-lipoic acid – all powerful antioxidants. The denser the colour, the higher the antioxidant content. Vibrant orange foods like apricots, calendula, carrots, mangoes, oranges, papaya, pumpkin, rockmelon, rosehip and sweet potato are rich in the major antioxidant beta-carotene. Brilliant red and pink foods like tomatoes, watermelon and pink grapefruit are wonderful sources of lycopene. Green and black tea are also rich in antioxidants.

ALPHA-HYDROXY ACIDS (AHAS) & FRUIT ENZYMES accelerate the skin's natural shedding process by dissolving the dead, flaking skin of the epidermis (outer layer of the skin) and exposing the newer and smoother skin underneath.

PROBIOTICS help to replenish, feed and and fortify the skin's microbiome, protecting the delicate skin barrier and subsequently fortifying our immune defences. Rich in naturally occurring alpha-hydroxy acids (AHAs), probiotics smooth, brighten and hydrate skin.

FATTY ACIDS plump up the skin cells, helping them retain moisture, and restore the barrier function of the skin. They are found in vegetable oils, seeds and nuts.

VITAMIN A helps improve the skin's elasticity and thickness, reduces the signs of photo-aging and is also very healing for acneous skin. It is found in apple, carrot seed oil, dandelion, egg yolks, milk, orange, rosehip oil, tomato and yoghurt.

VITAMIN C is a potent antioxidant that helps heal wounds, stimulate collagen and promote elastin, therefore improving skin's elasticity and tone and diminishing the appearance of fine lines and wrinkles. It also fights free radicals – triggered by sun exposure, pollution or stress – which can damage the skin. It's found in vegetables, herbs, grains, citrus fruits and some plant oils including rosehip oil.

VITAMIN E is an antioxidant and anti-inflammatory emollient that helps fight free radicals, soothes and smooths the skin, and aids in tissue healing. It's found naturally in vegetables, oils, nuts, seeds, whole grains, wheat flour and dairy products. Make sure you buy vitamin E in its natural form, tocopherol.

BUYING INGREDIENTS

Some of the ingredients used in my recipes are more readily available than others. Dried herbs and roots can be purchased at the supermarket or from a health food shop. Floral waters and clays can be bought at a health food shop or chemist, or from a supplier. Essential oils can be found in many retail shops, but your local health food store or chemist, or a supplier, may be your best bet. To ensure that you are buying the pure distilled essences and not dubious chemical concoctions, look for the botanical name on the bottle and buy from a reputable, well-established company that specialises in essential oils. If you are sensitive to essential oils, you can omit them from the recipes in this book – the recipes will still work without them. See page 172 for suppliers.

Opt for organic produce where possible. That way you can ensure your preparations are free of synthetic chemicals.

HYGIENE & STERILISATION

Good hygiene is an integral part of being a successful home cosmetician. Preparations contaminated with bacteria or mould can be harmful to the skin, especially when it is broken or cracked.

To keep your cosmetics pure and safe, follow these tips:

- Tie your hair back if it's long.
- Wear an apron.
- Wash your hands well, before and during preparation.
- Keep towels handy to dry your hands.
- Ensure your utensils are clean.
- Clean your chopping boards with salt before you begin.

To sterilise glass or plastic containers, put them in boiling water for 20 minutes, then leave them to dry completely, away from pollutants and contaminants. Make sure the water you use in your recipes is as pure as possible. If possible, use filtered water.

YOUR TOOLS

You will need some basic tools, most of which you may already have
in your kitchen. It is wise to keep some utensils separate from your
cooking tools. Wooden spoons, for example, absorb flavours and
smells – you don't want to end up with tea-tree–flavoured pancakes!
Some substances like beeswax are also difficult to clean off surfaces.
Here are some tools you might not already have:

- rubber spatulas
- measuring cups and spoons
- heat-resistant glass mixing bowls (Pyrex bowls are ideal)
- coffee filter papers
- mortar and pestle
- electric coffee grinder
- spray bottles
- pump bottles
- double boiler (bain-marie) or small saucepan with a Pyrex glass bowl
  that fits inside
- sensitive weighing scales
- glass dropper (for measuring essential oils and other small
  quantities) – also known as a pipette
- muslin (buy a metre-long piece and cut it into smaller square pieces)
- small and large funnels
- small battery-operated mixing wand
- two kitchen thermometers

Make sure that all your utensils are sterilised in boiling water. Do not
use metal bowls or spoons, as they oxidise with fruit and vegetable
juices and clay. Where possible, opt to use recycled glass jars or bottles
that you already have in your kitchen.

ALLERGIES

The recipes in this book contain natural, wholefood-based ingredients and although they are less likely to cause an allergic reaction, it is possible. If a reaction such as skin redness occurs, take off the preparation or mask immediately and rinse with lots of cold water. If it's an essential oil, remove it with a fatty oil such as olive or sweet almond oil. If you have sensitive skin, or are in any doubt, I recommend doing a patch test prior to application. To do this, simply apply one of the ingredients to a plaster and attach it firmly to the soft skin just inside your elbow. Leave it on for 24 hours and check for any reaction. If you have particularly sensitive skin, patch testing is important before applying any preparations to your face. To test essential oils, add 1 drop to 1 teaspoon of oil and leave for 24 hours. If there is no reaction, redness, soreness or itchiness, the ingredient is safe to use in your preparations. A reminder that oil preparations used in the shower can make the recess very slippery. So please be careful and wipe down afterwards.

VEGETABLE OILS, FATS & WAXES

Pure vegetable oils, fats and waxes are extracted from the seeds, kernels, nuts and other parts of plants. They are used widely in cosmetics to soften, smooth and moisturise skin and hair, and protect them from moisture loss. They are rich in essential fatty acids, antioxidants, vitamins and minerals, and provide effective, complementary bases for essential oils.

Vegetable oils are best extracted without heat (which destroys many of their nutritive qualities) so opt for unrefined, cold-pressed varieties. Most cold-pressed oils will last up to 9 months in the fridge – at cold temperatures they tend to go cloudy, which is a good sign that they are unrefined. When buying sesame oil make sure it's unrefined, not the darker variety often used in Asian cooking.

CLAYS

Argiletz (French) clays are cleansing, detoxifying, drawing, exfoliating, healing, soothing, toning and rejuvenating. They can be incorporated into cleansers, scrubs, masks, body powders, scalp treatments and bath preparations.

The depth at which active clays are extracted from the earth affects their active mineral content, colour and use. There are five different colours of Argiletz clay; each has properties suitable for a particular skin type. Green clay is the most absorbent and is suited to acneous, oily and neglected skin; pink clay is purifying and toning and suitable for all skin types; red clay helps treat sensitive skin and broken capillaries; white clay is the gentlest clay and it is soothing, softening and suitable for all skin types; and yellow clay is recommended for restoring tired and neglected skin of all types.

FLORAL WATERS

Floral waters are also known as waters of distillation, or hydrosols. They are the by-products of essential oil distillation. Floral waters help hydrate, tone, soothe, heal and freshen the skin and are wonderful in cosmetic preparations.

It is important to buy the authentic waters. For the recipes in this book, I have used chamomile water, lavender water, orange blossom water, rosewater and jasmine water. See pages 166–70 for skin types these floral waters are suited to.

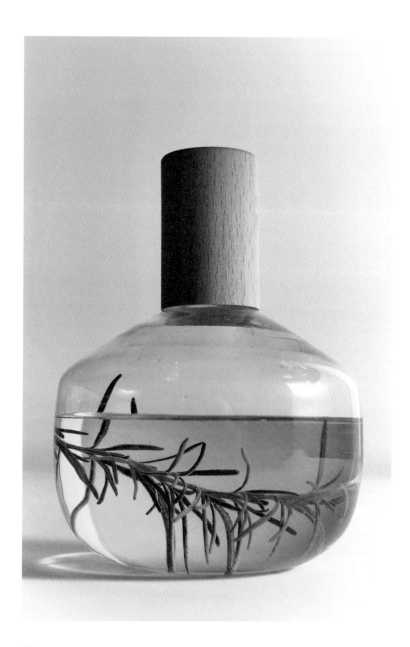

Aromatherapy

Essential oils work wonderfully in skincare, providing all the elements required for healthy skin function. The rejuvenating, antiseptic and toning properties of essential oils can help prevent or clear skin congestion and stimulate the generation of new cells. Because essential oils are made up of small molecules, they penetrate deep into the dermis. They also help balance our emotions through their wondrous scents. In fact, the emotional resonance of these oils is so powerful, it's very important that you like the scent of the oil for it to work optimally.

Essential oils can be incorporated into cleansers, creams, lotions, ointments, gels, toilette waters and perfumes. You can use them at 1 per cent dilution (around 20 drops in 5 tablespoons of a preparation). Essential oils alone or combined make beautiful therapeutic perfumes. The benefits of essential oils are that they:

- are highly antiseptic
- help speed up the removal of old skin cells and promote the growth of new skin cells
- improve muscle tone and blood circulation
- help eliminate waste
- reduce inflammation
- regulate sebum production, and
- reduce the impact of emotional stress.

PRECAUTIONS

Essential oils are highly concentrated forms of plant energy and can be harmful if not used properly; 1 drop of essential oil is said to have the therapeutic value of about 6 litres of herbal infusion. Do not take essential oils internally (unless prescribed by a practitioner) and keep them far away from children. Do not apply pure essential oils directly onto the skin and never exceed the recommended dose.

PREGNANCY & BREASTFEEDING

Many aromatherapists recommend that women avoid using some essential oils during pregnancy, especially in the first 3 months. You should always consult a qualified aromatherapist before using any aromatherapy products, even those you have made at home.

PHOTOSENSITIVITY

Certain essential oils can make the skin photosensitive, which means it is more prone to burning when exposed to ultraviolet light. These oils are: angelica root, bergamot, bitter orange, cold-pressed lime, grapefruit and lemon. It's best to avoid the sunlight for at least 12 hours after applying any of these oils, although they are fine in cleansers if washed off thoroughly. If you do wear them, be sure to apply an SPF.

SKIN IRRITATIONS

There are some oils which are more likely to irritate sensitive skin: basil, cinnamon leaf and bark, clove bud, lemon, lemongrass, tea-tree and thyme. Sensitivity varies from person to person and oil to oil.

PURE ESSENTIAL OIL COMPOSITIONS

Here are some suggestions for essential oil combinations for particular skin types. These quantities can be added to 5 tablespoons of base formula or oil.

NORMAL 10 drops lavender, 6 geranium, 4 ylang-ylang

OILY 8 drops sandalwood, 6 lemon, 6 lavender

DRY 8 drops sandalwood, 6 geranium, 6 rose

COMBINATION 10 drops lavender, 6 geranium, 4 orange

SENSITIVE 6 drops chamomile, 4 rose, 2 neroli

DEHYDRATED 10 drops rose, 8 sandalwood, 2 patchouli

MATURE 8 drops neroli, 6 frankincense, 6 ylang-ylang

ACNEOUS 10 drops lemon, 10 cypress, 5 lavender

DEVITALISED 10 drops geranium, 6 rose, 4 cypress

BROKEN CAPILLARIES 8 drops rose, 6 chamomile, 6 cypress

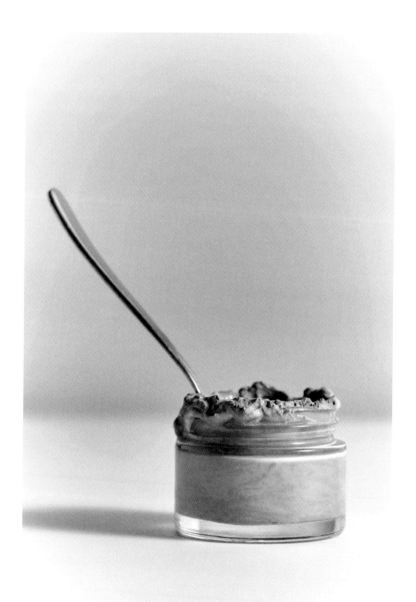

Preserving
your creations

Antimicrobial preservatives reduce the growth of bacteria and fungi in your preparations. Instead of using parabens and the formaldehyde-based preservatives found in many commercial cosmetics, look out for healthier alternatives like grapefruit seed extract (also known as citrus seed extract or citricidal). Grapefruit seed extract is an antimicrobial and fungicidal. Add at 0.5–3 per cent to water or herbal infusion.

To help prevent your vegetable and nut oils from oxidising, add an antioxidant, such as vitamin E. The vitamin E (tocopherol) oil should be 1–5 per cent of your total oil content, which is 1–5 ml (⅛ fl oz) per 100 ml (3½ fl oz). Or use amiox (rosemary extract or herbalox) at 0.1–0.5 per cent, which is approximately 2–10 drops per 100 ml (3½ fl oz).

LONGEVITY OF COSMETICS

- All long-life emulsions may last up to 6 months, especially if kept refrigerated.
- All dry scrubs, if kept dry, will last up to 3 months, especially if kept refrigerated.
- Any formulations containing alcohol will last up to 1 year.
- Treatment oils with amiox or vitamin E added should last 6 months.
- Balms should last up to 6 months.
- Herbal infusions or water-based products will last up to 3 days in the fridge without citrus seed extract Alternatively, freeze in ice cube trays to extend their lifespan.
- Fresh masks will last 1–2 days.

Base recipes

These recipes provide the basic methods you will need to make the preparations in the Face and Body sections. You can also use them as a starting point for creating your own recipes.

HERBAL PREPARATIONS

Dried herbs in dry preparations will keep, but once they are in the form of a decoction or infusion, they will only last a couple of days. Add up to 80 ml (2½ fl oz) vodka to the recipes in this section to prevent them from spoiling. Alternatively, freeze them in ice cube trays and use as required.

When making these preparations, avoid using metal pots and containers, as they may react with the herbs. Instead, use Pyrex, enamel or china vessels. To extract the active ingredients from the herbs, it's a good idea to pummel them first using a mortar and pestle.

If you are time-poor, you can use herbal tea bags instead of loose herbs.

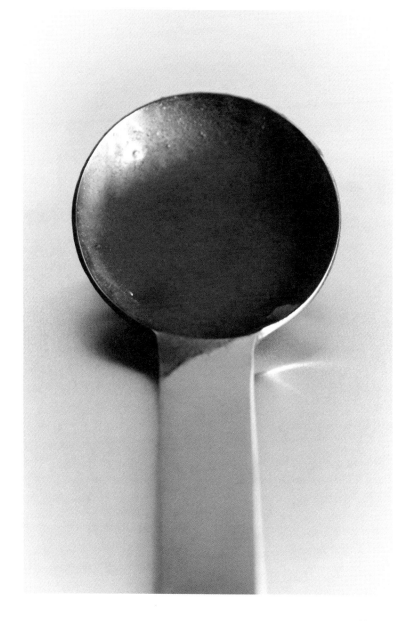

Infusions

Herbal infusions make wonderful remedial face washes and toners and can be incorporated into almost any preparation. The softer, more delicate parts of the plant (the flowers and leaves) are used. See pages 166–70 for which herbs suit your skin type.

> 2 teaspoons dried herb or 4 teaspoons fresh herb, finely chopped
> 250 ml (8½ fl oz/1 cup) boiling water

– Place the herb in a heat-resistant pitcher or bowl. Cover the herb with the boiling water and leave to steep for at least 15 minutes. Cover the pitcher or bowl to prevent the loss of volatile elements through evaporation.
– Strain the infusion.

Decoctions

To make a decoction, a herb is boiled gently in water to extract the active ingredients. The harder parts of the plant (the roots, rhizomes, bark, seeds and berries) are used. The resultant decoction can be used in the same way as an infusion.

> 2 teaspoons dried herb or 4 teaspoons fresh herb, chopped or crushed
> 375 ml (12½ fl oz/1½ cups) water

– Put the herb and water in a saucepan and bring to the boil.
– Cover tightly and simmer gently for 25 minutes.
– Strain and filter if necessary.

Vinegars

Herbal vinegars can be used as skin tonics, wound solutions, body splashes, deodorants, hair rinses and bath additives. Apple cider vinegar is an ideal base.

– Fill a jar with chopped fresh herbs or half-fill a jar with dried herbs, and pour in enough apple cider vinegar to fill the jar. Secure the lid.
– Leave the jar in a warm, protected place for 2 weeks and shake the bottle twice daily.
– Strain and filter, then bottle and store in a cool place, preferably the fridge.

Tinctures

Herbal tinctures, often referred to as 'mother tinctures', are stronger and more concentrated than infusions or decoctions and have a much longer shelf life. The minimum concentration of alcohol needed for preservation is 40 per cent of a preparation. You need to use an alcohol that is at least 60 per cent proof. Vodka is around this amount. Because alcohol is an excellent solvent for plant materials, tinctures have potent remedial and healing qualities.

30 g (1 oz) dried herb
250 ml (8½ fl oz/1 cup) vodka

– Place the herb in a jar and pour over the vodka.
– Seal the jar, leave in a cool place and shake twice daily for 2 weeks.
– Strain and filter through muslin (cheesecloth) and then through coffee filter paper.
– Store in a dark glass bottle.

Infused oils

A herbal-infused oil works well in creams, ointments, massage oils and bath oils. To make, you will need fresh herbs and a light, almost odourless, cold-pressed vegetable oil such as jojoba, sweet almond or apricot kernel oil.

– Fill a jar with freshly chopped herbs and/or flowers. If only using herbs, half-fill the jar.
– Cover the herbs with vegetable oil until the jar is full.
– Seal the jar, leave in a warm place for 2 weeks (not in direct sunlight or the oil will become rancid) and shake twice daily. Delicate flowers like jasmine and honeysuckle decompose quickly, so it's important to replace them daily.
– Strain through muslin (cheesecloth). Pour into a jar and store in the fridge.
– After a few days, carefully decant the oil into a glass bottle, leaving the sediment behind. Refrigerate.

Ointments & balms

Ointments, balms and salves are made from oils, waxes and fats and have no water content. They are thick and buttery, combine well with herbs and essential oils, and are used to help heal dry, irritated skin. They provide the skin with more protection than normal moisturisers, as they stay on the surface of the skin longer, making them ideal for treating chapped lips and nappy rash (but they should not be left on excessively oily skin). Jars of ointment will keep for months in the fridge, and make superb gifts.

Beeswax, cocoa butter, vegetable oils and shea butter are the basic ingredients. Sweet almond oil, apricot oil and jojoba oil are ideal vegetable oils, as they remain relatively stable when heated.

3–5 tablespoons vegetable oil
15 g (½ oz) beeswax
10 g (¼ oz) cocoa butter

OINTMENT METHOD 1 – USING HERBS
– Place 30–50 g (1–1¾ oz) of dried or 90–150 g (3–5½ oz) of fresh herb with the oil in a bain-marie. Heat over a low heat until the herb loses its normal colour.
– Strain and allow to cool.
– Melt the beeswax and cocoa butter in a bain-marie over low heat.
– Remove from the heat and add the herbal oil, mixing well.
– Pour into glass jars and store in the fridge.

OINTMENT METHOD 2 – USING HERBAL TINCTURES
– Place the oil, beeswax and cocoa butter in a bain-marie. Warm over a low heat until the beeswax and cocoa butter have melted.
– Add 2 teaspoons of a herbal tincture, mixing thoroughly.
– Pour into glass jars and store in the fridge.

OINTMENT METHOD 3 – USING FINELY GROUND DRIED HERB
– Melt the oil, beeswax and cocoa butter in a bain-marie.
– Stir in 1–3 tablespoons of finely ground dried herb and simmer
  for 20 minutes.
– Strain through muslin (cheesecloth), then coffee filter paper.
  Pour into glass jars and store in the fridge.

OINTMENT METHOD 4 – USING HERBAL-INFUSED OIL
– Melt the beeswax, cocoa butter and the infused oil (instead of the
  vegetable oil) in a bain-marie and mix thoroughly.
– Warm over a low heat until the beeswax and cocoa butter have melted.
  Mix thoroughly.
– Pour into glass jars and store in the fridge.

MAYONNAISES

A mayonnaise made from fresh organic eggs, cold-pressed vegetable
oils and aromatic essential oils is a sumptuous feast for thirsty skin and
hair. This type of mayonnaise makes an easy, inexpensive, luxurious
and convenient face and body cleanser, moisturiser, bath cream or
hair treatment. You can use any high-quality oil, although you should
choose one to suit your skin type (pages 166–70). A batch will last for
2–3 weeks in the fridge. Measure your drops of essential oil with
a plastic pipette.

> 1 egg yolk
> 250 ml (8½ fl oz/1 cup) cold-pressed vegetable oil
> 1 teaspoon honey
> ½ teaspoon apple cider vinegar
> 20 drops essential oil (optional – vanilla oil is lovely in this recipe)

– Beat the egg yolk in a blender.
– Slowly pour in the vegetable oil and continue mixing until the noise
  of the blender changes; this is a sign the mixture is getting thicker.
– Slowly add the remaining ingredients, in order, mixing until well combined.
– Store in a glass jar in the fridge.

PLANT GELS

Gel formulations are very hydrating and soothing. They make good oil-free cleansers, moisturisers and masks, eye treatments and hair gels, and are particularly useful in the warmer months when skin becomes greasier. Gels can be made from myriad foods; those most commonly used are linseeds, pectin (from citrus peel), guar gum, xanthan gum, arrowroot, Irish moss, marshmallow root, agar-agar and tapioca. Aloe vera gel is also a suitable gel base.

Plant gels are made by adding water to pectin, guar or xanthan gum. They will last up to one week in an airtight jar in the fridge.

Basic plant gel

This gel can be used as a moisturiser, eye gel or mask.

5 tablespoons purified water or floral water
½–3 teaspoons powdered pectin or xanthan gum or guar gum (depending on the desired consistency)
10 drops essential oil

- Warm the water or floral water over a medium heat (do not boil) then remove from heat.
- Slowly sprinkle the powdered gum into the water or floral water and whisk until the desired consistency is reached.
- To make the gel smooth, push it through a strainer. If it is too thick for your liking, add more water.
- Add the essential oil and mix well.
- Store in a glass jar in the fridge.

Linseed gel

Linseed gel is emollient and very soothing. It is an excellent first aid gel for bruises, sprains, swellings, inflammations and burns. It also makes an impressive soothing, calming and plumping mask.

2 tablespoons linseeds
250 ml (8½ fl oz/1 cup) boiling water or herbal infusion

- Simmer the linseeds in the boiling water or herbal infusion until a gel forms.
- Strain the seeds from the gel, retaining the water or herbal infusion. Dilute the gel with the strained water or herbal infusion if a thinner consistency is desired.
- Store in a glass jar in the fridge.

EMULSIONS

Oil and water don't mix. However, with the use of an emulsifier, they can be bound together to form milky or creamy mixtures called 'emulsions'. Mayonnaise is an example of an emulsion; in mayonnaise the ingredient (the emulsifier) that binds the oil and vinegar together in a consistent form is the egg yolk. Without an emulsifier, you would end up with a mixture similar to salad dressing, where the vinegar sits buoyantly on top of the oil.

Most commercial cleansers and moisturisers are emulsions, and emulsions are the most complex preparations in this book. The secret? It's all in the way you mix. Depending on what goes together and how it is mixed, you can end up with either an omelette or a soufflé! But with practise, it becomes very easy and you can make a year's supply of face cream within an hour.

There are two types of emulsion. The first is an oil-in-water emulsion, which contains mostly water. Emulsions in this group include cleansing milks, cleansing creams, face creams and body lotions. The second type is a water-in-oil emulsion, which contains mostly oil. These emulsions feel thicker and greasier on the skin and include cold creams, ointments and barrier creams.

When an emulsion is made, two phases – the oil phase and the water phase – are required. In both phases, the ingredients are heated. Once the desired temperature is reached, the products of the two phases are combined to form the emulsion.

You can add your desired combination of pure essential oils, infused oils, cold-pressed vegetable oils, floral waters, herbal infusions and herbal tinctures. See pages 166–70 for ingredients to suit your skin type. Measure your drops of essential oils and preservatives with plastic pipettes.

Emulsion

For 100 g (3½ oz)

OIL PHASE
8 g (¼ oz) plant-derived emulsifying wax (plus other solid fats, as given in individual recipes)
20 ml (¾ fl oz) vegetable oil or infused oil
4 drops rosemary leaf extract

WATER PHASE
75 ml (2½ fl oz) purified or demineralised water
1 teaspoon vegetable glycerine
15 drops grapefruit seed extract

THIRD PHASE
20 drops essential oil suited to your skin type (see pages 166–70)

– Melt the waxes (and other solid fats) and the vegetable or infused oil (unless the oil is high in fatty acids, such as avocado, evening primrose, linseed or rosehip oil, which deteriorate if exposed to high heat for too long, in which case it should be added at the next stage) in a bain-marie over a medium heat, stirring occasionally until well mixed.
– Remove from the heat and add any vegetable oils high in fatty acids and the rosemary leaf extract to the heated oils and waxes. At 65°C, your mix is ready for the water phase.
– Heat the combined water, glycerine and grapefruit seed extract to 65°C then slowly add to the oil phase over a low heat, mixing continuously using a small hand-held mixing wand.
– Remove from the heat. The emulsion will be very watery in consistency and look milky.

- Continue mixing (oil-in-water emulsions can separate, so stir briskly) for a short time (about 20 seconds at the most). If the mixture does separate, simply remix it. Keep stirring by hand until the mixture starts to thicken and cool. Water-in-oil emulsions need to be stirred slowly and steadily.
- When the emulsion has cooled a little, add the essential oils (third phase).
- Pour into small jars.

AROMATHERAPY OINTMENTS & BALMS

Aromatherapy ointments and balms can be used as massage balms, healing ointments and perfume balms.

15 g (½ oz) beeswax
10 g (¼ oz) cocoa butter
3–5 tablespoons cold-pressed vegetable oil (and/or shea butter)
20–40 drops essential oil (add more or less depending on desired strength)

- Melt the beeswax and cocoa butter with the vegetable oil or shea butter in a bain-marie, then remove from heat.
- When the mixture starts to cool, add the essential oils and mix thoroughly.
- Pour into glass jars.

Face

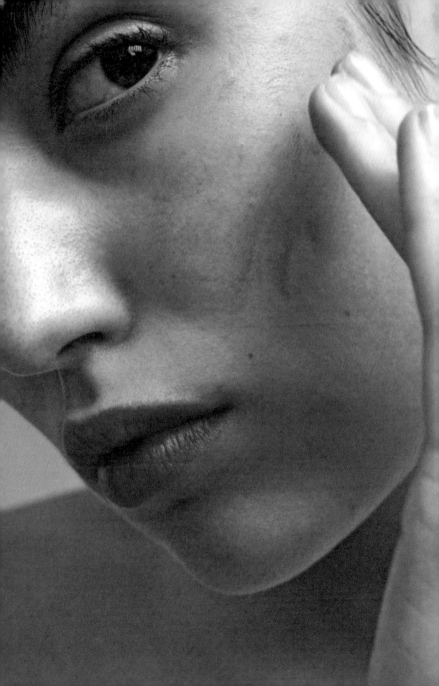

Cleansers

I must confess that a few splashes of water over a night-out's worth of dirt and makeup have often left me kidding myself that I've cleaned my face. But skin is too smart for such play. By the following morning, without fail, my skin has retaliated with a generous outburst of spots. As tempting as it may be, cleansing should never be a slapdash affair. It is the first and most important step in your skincare ritual, gently removing excess oil, makeup, pollution, grit and grime accumulated during the day. It also helps loosen dead skin cells, dislodge blackheads and clean out pores. Poorly cleansed skin leaves oil glands congested with dirt and cellular waste, which is the perfect environment for unwanted breakouts.

The following recipes are free from surfactants, which are often found in many (but not all) commercial cleansers. Some common surfactants, like sodium lauryl sulfate, strip the skin of its natural oils and upset its pH. This can often irritate the skin and send oil glands into overdrive, making oily skin even slicker. Soapy suds and big foamy bubbles may be impressive, but they do not clean better than other, milder cleansers; they just indicate a harsh product. Commercial soaps are also harsh, and can leave skin feeling parched, tight and uncomfortable. When shopping for cleansers, if you're not making your own, make sure to read the label if you wish to avoid such ingredients.

Forming the habit of properly cleansing your face not only removes all kinds of dirt from the surface of the skin, but also prepares your face to better absorb the nutrients in the products you use. To cleanse properly, gently press the face with a warm, damp soft cloth to help loosen clogged pores and soften surface cells. Apply your cleanser using sparklingly clean hands, a cotton cloth or resuable cotton pads, depending on the cleanser used. If using your hands, massage the cleanser into the face and neck using an upward circular motion, pressing along the main meridians of the face and neck and behind the ears. This facilitates the flow of oxygen-carrying blood to the face, enhancing the tone and texture of the complexion.

To remove cleanser, always use a cotton cloth or face washer – as splashing water from cupped hands will not lift surface grime. Muslin (cheesecloth) wash cloths are my favourite medium for removing cleansers, as they gently exfoliate the skin and wipe away the residue. Take your time and when finished, rinse your cloth thoroughly and hang to dry. Replace every two days with a fresh, clean cloth. And if you have time, cleanse twice: once to remove surface dirt and makeup and a second time to get the skin really clean.

As the seasons change, so too will your cleanser requirements. In colder months, you may need a richer, more nourishing cleanser than in summer, when skin produces more oil. During a stressful patch, your skin may become sensitive or dehydrated and require a different cleanser to cater for and help remedy the imbalance.

Use your cleanser twice daily: once lightly in the morning to remove waste the skin has expelled overnight and once in the evening to wash away the day's collection of dirt.

FERMENTED MILK & CREAM CLEANSERS

Milk has been used for centuries as a natural cleanser, but for some, dairy milk can cause allergic reactions. Where possible, opt for fermented varieties such as kefir – which are naturally rich in probiotic bacteria and replete with acids, lipids and enzymes, which help remove dead skin cells, prevent blackheads and smooth the skin. Natural yoghurt or buttermilk also works well for all skin types, especially oily and untoned, while goat's milk, buttermilk and soy milk are kind on more sensitive skins. These milk cleansers can be used alone or with herbs and essential oils. Store in an airtight bottle in the fridge for up to 1 week.

Apply with a reusable cotton makeup pad or cloth in upward, circular motions, then rinse with lots of tepid water and a clean cloth or face washer. I prefer to use a milk cleanser in the morning and something a little more rigorous in the evening.

Brightening kefir cleanser
For dull, devitalised skin

Kefir is rich beneficial bacteria that helps to balance the skin as well as enzymes that help to deeply cleanse and brighten the complexion.

    2 tablespoons dairy or coconut kefir
    ¼ teaspoon lemon or lime juice

– Mix the kefir and lime juice thoroughly.

Honey cream cleanser
For all skin types

This mildly astringent cleanser will cleanse, tone and smooth. It is especially useful for skin that needs a lift.

    1 teaspoon honey
    1 teaspoon natural yoghurt

– In a small bowl, thoroughly combine the honey and yoghurt (you may need to warm the honey first).
– Apply to damp skin with hands, then rinse your skin 3 times with a damp, tepid cloth and pat dry with a soft towel.

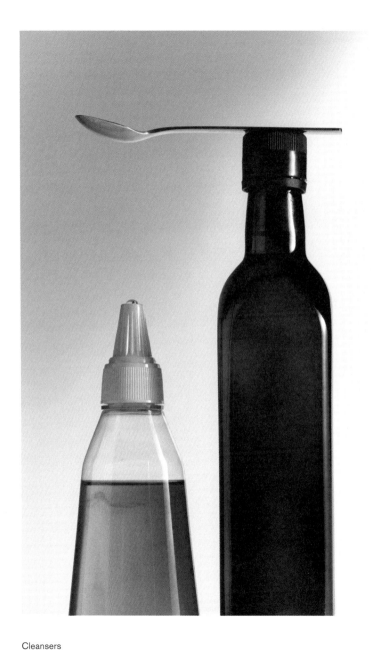

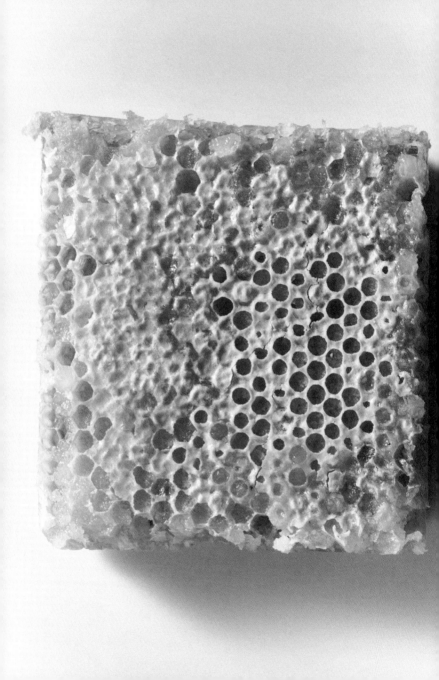

CLEANSING OILS

Cleansing oils have been used in various cultures for centuries and are still very popular in the Middle East. Unrefined, cold-pressed vegetable and nut oils are superb skin cleansers. Unlike the mineral oils that are often found in commercial cleansers, they don't just sit on the skin, but dissolve impurities on the surface of the skin while feeding it with nutrients.

As strange as it may sound, cleansing oily skin with oil is very effective. With the oil layered onto the skin, the sebaceous glands are tricked into thinking they have produced enough oil and don't make more. Light oils like jojoba, hazelnut, sweet almond and apricot kernel are ideal for oily skin. The base oils I recommend for all skin types are jojoba, sweet almond, apricot kernel, sesame, sunflower and grape seed. Small percentages of heavier oils like avocado and wheat germ can be added for drier, more mature skin. Cleansing oils should be applied to a damp face and massaged over the face and neck, then removed with a damp face washer and lots of tepid water. Your oil cleanser will last up to 6 months in a cool dark place. Add the contents of 2 vitamin E capsules to help preserve. Follow with a toner.

Queen bee oil cleanser
For all skin types

A mix of honey and almond oil makes an excellent facial cleanser that lifts stubborn city grime.

½ teaspoon honey
½ teaspoon sweet almond oil

– Mix the honey into the sweet almond oil (you may need to warm the honey first). Make fresh as needed.

Illuminating oil cleanser

Coconut oil is both nourishing as well as being anti-fungal and anti-microbial, making it the perfect cleanser for all skin types. It leaves the skin feeling both soft and glowing.

2½ tablespoons coconut oil (room temperature)
2½ tablespoons apricot kernel oil
10 drops lime essential oil

– Combine the oils thoroughly. Store in a well-sealed glass bottle.

Sweet dreams cleansing oil
For all skin types

This cleanser has good antimicrobial action and an uplifting scent. I often use it in the evening, when my skin feels like it is carrying the weight of the world.

4 tablespoons sweet almond oil
3 tablespoons sunflower oil
1 teaspoon vitamin E oil
7 drops mandarin essential oil
6 drops sandalwood essential oil
5 drops lavender essential oil
2 drops lemon essential oil

– Combine the oils thoroughly. Store in a well-sealed glass bottle.

Sticky butter cleansing balm
For all skin types

I'd never considered making a cleansing/exfoliating balm until I had the pleasure of experiencing how delicious they could feel when a facialist used one on my skin for the first time many years ago. After a few experiments and iterations, I came up with this wonder balm. The key is to wipe the luscious, sticky balm away with warm water and a cotton cloth at least 3 times to remove thoroughly. Finish skin with a toner to eliminate excess grease.

20 g (¾ oz) cocoa butter

12 g (½ oz) beeswax

4 tablespoons sweet almond oil

1 teaspoon honey

8 drops rosemary leaf extract

2 drops eucalyptus essential oil

2 drops peppermint essential oil

20 drops grapefruit essential oil

10 drops hops essential oil

– Slowly melt the cocoa butter, wax, oil and honey in a bain-marie, stirring gently. Once melted, take off the heat.
– When the mixture has cooled to body temperature, add the essential oils and rosemary leaf extract. Mix thoroughly.
– Pour into jars.
– Gently massage a small amount into the skin for a couple of minutes. Using a soft muslin cloth, or cotton face washer, and a sink full of tepid water, patting and pressing your face with the cloth, wipe away the balm. Wipe and rinse in this way three times. This balm will last up to six months.

OAT CLEANSERS

Oats are remarkably cleansing, healing, anti-inflammatory, softening and moisturising. They are also high in silica and therefore great for skin, nails and hair. For years, professionals have heralded oats as the healing grain, recommending them for irritated and sensitive skin. Keep a jar of fine oatmeal near your sink, in the shower and bath, and use to cleanse every inch of your body. Add a couple of drops of lavender essential oil to each container to make the oats fragrant. Wrap a handful of oats in a piece of muslin (cheesecloth) and use as a wash balloon for babies' tender skin. They will love it!

Almond milk or oat milk paste cleanser
For all skin types

Soak almond meal or oatmeal overnight in a milk suited to your skin type (pages 166–70) and use the mix to cleanse your face in the morning. Both combinations are very cleansing and hydrating, and will keep the skin blemish-free.

LONG-LIFE EMULSION CLEANSERS

Mandarin & ylang–ylang milk cleanser

For all skin types

You can alter the essential oils for a light and fragrant cleanser to suit your skin type (pages 166–70).

OIL PHASE
7 g (¼ oz) plant-derived emulsifying wax
15 ml (½ fl oz) apricot kernel oil
5 drops rosemary leaf extract

WATER PHASE
80 ml (2½ fl oz) purified water or floral water
14 drops grapefruit seed extract

THIRD PHASE
12 drops mandarin essential oil
8 drops ylang-ylang essential oil

– Follow the instructions for making an emulsion on page 38.

Ultra–calming cleansing cream

For mature and very dry skin

This rich, grounding cream is also ideal for parched winter skin.

OIL PHASE
8 g (¼ oz) plant-derived emulsifying wax
2 g cocoa butter
15 ml (½ fl oz) sweet almond oil
5 ml (⅛ fl oz) honey
6 drops rosemary leaf extract

WATER PHASE
70 ml (2¼ fl oz) rosewater or purified water
15 drops grapefruit seed extract

THIRD PHASE
20 drops sandalwood essential oil

– Follow the instructions for making an emulsion on page 38.

FOAMING CLEANSERS

Castile soap is unlike other soaps, which often strip the skin of its natural oils. It is readily available at health food shops and offers a very gentle way to cleanse the face. You can adapt it by adding other ingredients to suit your skin type. Mixed with vegetable and nut oils, these cleansers produce a smooth, creamy, non-drying lather. The essential oils make these cleansers beautifully fragrant and enhance their cleansing, soothing and antibacterial properties. These cleansers will last up to 6 months stored in a glass jar in the fridge.

To use a foaming cleanser, apply a small amount to your fingertips, lather and apply to a damp face. Massage in upward circular motions. Remove with a cotton cloth and lots of tepid water.

Gentle Castile cleansing wash
For all skin types

In winter, when your skin is very dry, you may want to up the oil component to 1 tablespoon.

4½ tablespoons liquid Castile soap
2 teaspoons sweet almond or apricot kernel oil
20 drops essential oil suited to your skin type (pages 166–70)

– Pour or drop all the ingredients into a bottle and shake well.

Soapwort cleanser
For sensitive skin and skin with eczema

Soapwort is one of the gentlest ways to cleanse very sensitive skin. It contains natural saponins, which create an impressive lather.

1 tablespoon soapwort root, chopped and bruised
375 ml (12½ fl oz/1½ cups) water
1 teaspoon dried red clover or calendula flowers

– Mix the herbs and water together in a small saucepan. Bring to the boil.
– Simmer gently over a low heat for 15 minutes.
– Remove from the heat, allow to cool, then strain and bottle. To thicken, add a little citrus pectin or xanthan gum.
– Use within 3–4 days or freeze in ice cube trays for later use.

Geranium & clay cleanser

For oily and acneous skin

Jojoba is one of the best oils for acne-prone skin as it helps to balance the skin and sebum production.

20 drops geranium essential oil

2 teaspoons jojoba oil

4 tablespoons liquid Castile soap

2 teaspoons green clay

– Add the essential oil and jojoba oil to the Castile soap and mix well.
– Mix in the clay well, smoothing out any clumps.

Lime & cedarwood cleansing/shaving oil

For all skin types

My husband swears by this recipe.

2½ tablespoons apricot kernel oil

2½ tablespoons liquid Castile soap

6 drops lime essential oil

4 drops atlas cedarwood essential oil

– Pour or drop all the ingredients into a bottle and shake well.
– Always shake before use. Apply to warm, damp skin before shaving.

Toners

Toners are refreshing elixirs applied to the skin after cleansing or masking to help remove or dissolve any residue. They are also used to help stimulate circulation, restore the skin's acid mantle, hydrate and refine the skin, and may help to reduce pore size. Avoid alcohol-based toners, which strip the skin of its natural oils, overstimulating the sebaceous glands and making your skin far greasier than before. The ideal toner should heal while correcting the skin's balance.

Apply with a resuable cotton pad or cloth after cleansing, in gentle, circular, upward motions. Leave on and follow with a moisturiser or lotion to suit your skin type.

ALOE VERA JUICE is an ideal toner for all skin types because of its astringent, antiseptic, healing and regenerative properties.

FLORAL WATERS make soothing and healing skin toners alone or as bases for other ingredients. They are especially suited to very sensitive skin.

HERBAL INFUSIONS make great toners. Choose herbs suited to your skin type (pages 166–70).

HERBAL VINEGARS make very effective toners. The vinegar helps restore the skin's pH and the herbs are cleansing, bracing and healing. To make, dilute 1 tablespoon (page 32) in 5 tablespoons of purified or floral water.

APPLE CIDER VINEGAR is naturally antimicrobal and can help restore the skin's natural pH making it an effective toner, especially for acne-prone skin. Mix one part apple cider vinegar with two parts filtered water.

RICE WATER TONER works well for sensitive and irritated skin types and helps to soothe conditions such as eczema. Simply soak ½ cup of cooked rice in 2–3 cups of water for 30 minutes before straining. Store in the fridge.

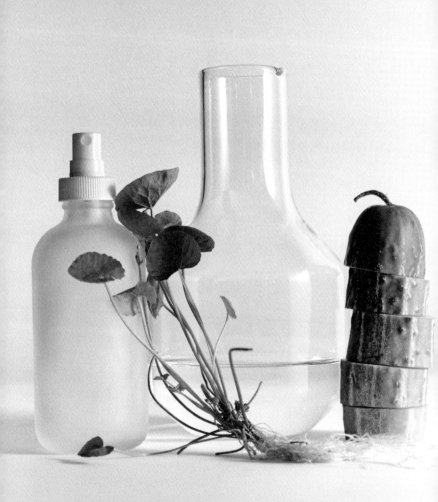

HERBAL INFUSIONS AND TONERS

The following herbal infusions are best made fresh, unless otherwise stated. Grapefruit seed extract will prolong their life span only a little, because of its high water content. It is just as easy to make these toners fresh every 7–10 days, storing them in glass bottles in the fridge. Or you can freeze batches in ice cube trays and thaw as needed. If short on time, you can use tea bags soaked in hot water as infusions.

Green tea & peppermint toner

For all skin types

Green tea is high in antioxidants and protects the skin from damage from free radicals. It is helpful for all skin types.

$2\frac{1}{2}$ tablespoons green tea infusion
$2\frac{1}{2}$ tablespoons peppermint infusion

– Mix the infusions, bottle and store in fridge.

Healing floral toner

For all skin types, especially sensitive and dehydrated

This very fragrant, healing toner is one of my favourites. Use a floral water to suit your skin type (pages 166–70). This toner will last for a few months in the fridge because of the addition of grapefruit seed extract.

$4\frac{1}{2}$ tablespoons floral water
2 teaspoons aloe vera juice
10 drops grapefruit seed extract

– Combine the ingredients, place in a glass jar and store in the fridge.

Elderflower water

For all skin types, especially oily skin with large pores or pigmentation

Elderflowers cleanse, tone and brighten the skin, and reduce pore size. Make a simple infusion of elderflowers (page 32), bottle and refrigerate.

Honey & lavender toner

For all skin types, especially oily and congested

This is a lovely healing and bracing toner.

¼ teaspoon honey
4 tablespoons witch hazel water
4 drops lavender essential oil
½ teaspoon apple cider vinegar

– Dissolve the honey in the witch hazel water.
– Add the essential oil to the apple cider vinegar, then add to the honey water. Store in the fridge for up to three months. Shake well before each use.

Parsley & ginseng tea toner

For mature and devitalised skin

Parsley is high in vitamin C and ginseng promotes skin elasticity and epidermal cell production. This is sure to bring back colour to your cheeks!

2½ tablespoons parsley infusion
2½ tablespoons ginseng decoction

– Mix the infusions well, bottle and refrigerate.

Orange & fennel toner

For lined and untoned skin

Fennel seeds and fennel essential oil contain phytoestrogens, which are plant-based compounds that firm and rejuvenate the skin by stimulating the metabolism of cells that make up the dermis. This lovely balancing, rejuvenating and fragrant toner is especially good for sluggish, untoned, lined skin, whether oily or dry.

½ teaspoon fennel seeds
5 tablespoons boiling water
2 teaspoons orange juice

– Crush the fennel seeds using a mortar and pestle. Pour the boiling water over the seeds and leave covered for 20 minutes.
– Strain the infusion, mix with the juice and bottle.

Basil & lemongrass toner

For blemished skin

An infusion of basil leaves (page 32) makes a cleansing and toning freshener. Basil can help acne sufferers by killing bacteria on the skin. The scent of basil is also a known antidepressant, making it especially useful if you're feeling a little glum about your complexion. Lemongrass has impressive astringent properties and helps normalise the action of the oil glands.

2½ tablespoons basil infusion
2½ tablespoons lemongrass infusion

– Mix the infusions together, bottle and store in the fridge.

Calming chamomile water

For sensitive and combination skin

Chamomile has remarkable antiseptic and soothing qualities. The apple juice helps refine the skin.

4 tablespoons chamomile infusion
1 tablespoon apple juice

– Mix the infusion with the juice, bottle and store in the fridge.

Jasmine & rose toner

For sensitive, mature and dehydrated skin

This gentle and beautifully scented toner also makes a lovely perfumed body spray. If you buy the floral waters from a supplier already preserved, this will last up to 6 months.

2½ tablespoons jasmine water
2½ tablespoons rosewater

– Mix the floral waters well. Bottle and store in the fridge.

Ceramide rice toner

For dull, mature skin

Rice water contains ceramides that firm and protect the skin and other compounds that brighten the skin and help even out skin tone.

2 cups uncooked rice
4 cups water

– Add rice and water into a bowl.
– Cover the bowl and leave in a cool, dark area overnight for 8–10 hours.
– After the rice has soaked and is foggy in colour, strain the rice water into a bottle. The preparation will last up to five days in the fridge.

Spirit soother toner

For all skin types

A simple infusion of witch hazel makes an excellent cosmetic. It is high in tannic acid, a soothing and refreshing astringent, and can help reduce broken thread veins and large pores. It is also antiseptic and can quickly reduce any kind of eye, face or body puffiness, which is why the American Native Peoples have used it for hundreds of years to reduce swelling from wounds.

Cucumber & gotu kola toner

For sensitive skin

This soothing, calming and brightening toner is especially beneficial for irritated and inflamed skin and for fine surface capillaries.

½ cucumber, peeled
3 tablespoons gotu kola infusion

– Juice the cucumber and strain.
– Mix the juice with the infusion, bottle and store in the fridge.

Treatment oils

Facial oils can be used to help regenerate and boost the skin, while also treating a specific condition. Facial oils that combine cold-pressed vegetable oils and essential oils activates the skin to replenish, heal, cleanse and tone.

Treatment oils can be used intermittently until the problem abates. Apply at night after cleansing and toning. If in the depths of winter your skin is feeling parched, you may want to apply and massage a fine layer of moisturiser into the skin, over the oil. If your skin is acneous, use a few drops mixed with water and don't give up – you may have to apply nightly for at least 1–2 weeks before you see any results. An intensive treatment with toning oils used at regular intervals is very beneficial for mature skin and can be used every night on an ongoing basis.

For facial oils use a 1 per cent dilution (20 drops in 5 tablespoons of base oil) of essential oils. Use only 0.25 per cent dilution (5 drops in 5 tablespoons) if using long-term, to prevent the skin from becoming sensitised to a particular oil.

Pour the oils into a bottle and shake until well blended.

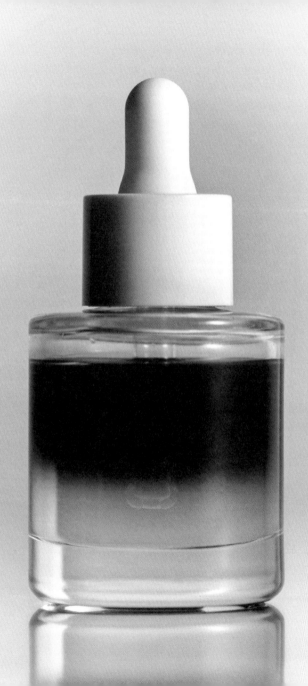

OIL COMBINATIONS

OILY SKIN 5 teaspoons hazelnut oil, 5 teaspoons jojoba oil, 4 drops sandalwood essential oil, 3 mandarin, 3 palmarosa

DRY SKIN 1 tablespoon sweet almond oil, 2 teaspoons avocado oil, 2 teaspoons olive oil, 2 teaspoons wheat germ oil, 4 drops sandalwood essential oil, 3 geranium, 3 rose

COMBINATION SKIN 5 teaspoons jojoba oil, 5 teaspoons sweet almond oil, 10 drops lavender essential oil, 6 geranium, 4 neroli

SENSITIVE SKIN (ECZEMA AND DERMATITIS) 5 teaspoons apricot kernel oil, 5 teaspoons jojoba oil, 3 drops chamomile essential oil, 3 atlas cedarwood, 2 lavender, 2 patchouli

DEHYDRATED SKIN $1\frac{1}{2}$ tablespoons apricot kernel oil, 1 tablespoon jojoba oil, 5 drops rose essential oil, 3 sandalwood, 2 palmarosa

MATURE SKIN 1 tablespoon jojoba oil, 2 teaspoons carrot root infused oil, 2 teaspoons evening primrose oil, 2 teaspoons rosehip oil, 6 drops rose essential oil, 3 frankincense, 2 patchouli

ACNEOUS SKIN $2\frac{1}{2}$ tablespoons apricot kernel oil, 1 tablespoon jojoba oil, 2 teaspoons borage seed oil, 4 drops carrot seed essential oil, 2 chamomile, 2 lavender, 2 tea-tree

ACNE SCARS $1\frac{1}{2}$ tablespoons jojoba oil, 2 teaspoons rosehip oil, 2 teaspoons wheat germ oil, 6 drops sandalwood essential oil, 4 lavender, 4 neroli

DEVITALISED SKIN 2 tablespoons apricot kernel oil, 2 teaspoons wheat germ oil, 5 drops geranium essential oil, 3 rose, 2 cypress

BROKEN CAPILLARIES 5 teaspoons apricot kernel oil, 5 teaspoons jojoba oil, 4 drops rose essential oil, 3 chamomile, 3 cypress

PIGMENTATION $1\frac{1}{2}$ tablespoons calendula-infused oil, 1 tablespoon rosehip oil, 5 drops celery essential oil, 5 lavender, 5 lovage

Moisturisers

Moisturisers help prevent dehydration and dryness while creating a protective barrier against free radicals and moisture loss. Homemade moisturisers created with the rich and nourishing oils of fruits, nuts, seeds, vegetables, natural waxes, healing herbs and therapeutic essential oils are not only luxurious treats that replenish, heal and revitalise skin – but they also help to nourish the skin microbiome and strengthen the skin's natural barrier function. The result? Calm, plump and juicy skin.

Moisturisers must contain both oil and water to keep the skin's surface layers soft and supple, and it is also important that they contain both emollients and humectants. Emollients – such as fat and oils – lock in moisture already present in the skin. Humectants attract water from the skin and the air and hold moisture in your cream and on your skin. A widely used humectant is glycerine, but honey is also effective. Ingredients best avoided are mineral oils and petroleum jelly. Although they remove makeup, they sit on the skin and cause pimples. They also have no nutritional value, only robbing skin of its precious fat-soluble vitamins. A light cream replete with nutritious and readily absorbed ingredients is ideal.

Moisturising in the morning after cleansing and toning is important to help protect the skin from the vicissitudes of daily life and should always be followed by an SPF. But it's also important to moisturise in the evening as our skin replenishes itself as we sleep. If you have particularly dehydrated skin, using a heavier cream at night can be beneficial, helping to lock in moisture. Apply your moisturiser to a damp face and massage it in well. If there is any remaining moisturiser after 15 minutes, pat dry.

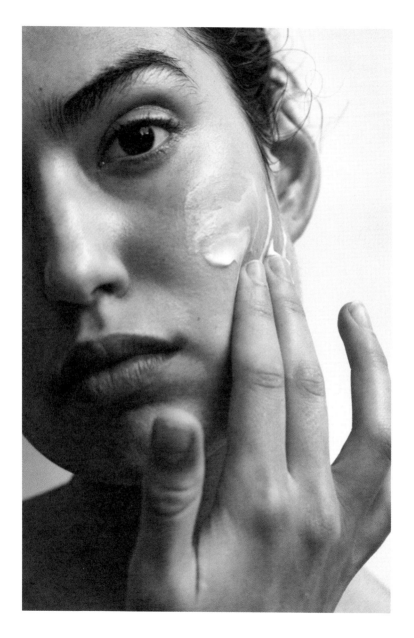

FRESH MILK LOTIONS

Milk is a natural emulsion saturated with enzymes, vitamins, minerals and lipids – and as mentioned earlier, fermented varieties like kefir boast further benefits as they are naturally rich in probiotic bacteria. Milk often comforts the skin naturally by increasing and retaining moisture levels, giving the complexion a smooth, creamy feel. These recipes are perfect for nighttime use, unless your skin is very dry. Simply apply with a reusable cotton makeup pad after cleansing and toning, and sleep on it. In the morning, your skin will feel super soft and supple.

Sleepy time probiotic lotion
For all skin types, especially dull and devitalised

Kefir contains enzymes and probiotics that help to balance your skin microbiome while you sleep. The addition of lavender oil will help inspire a relaxed sleep.

> 2 tespoons kefir
> ⅛ teaspoon honey
> 1 drop lavender essential oil (optional)

– Mix ingredients thoroughly.

Fresh cream moisturiser
For mature, dry skin

This rich moisturiser contains nourishing fats and refining acids that help to rejuvenate the skin, leaving it feeling soft and supple.

> 1 teaspoon fresh cream
> 1 drop rose geranium essential oil (optional)

– Mix ingredients thoroughly.

JOJOBA MOISTURISERS

Jojoba moisturising oil
For all skin types

The jojoba desert plant retains water during the long summer drought, and its waxy oil, pressed from the bean, does exactly that when applied to our skin. It provides a protective film over the skin and hair shaft, helping keep moisture in and free radicals out. Jojoba oil is very special and clever, and could almost be the extent of your beauty regimen – what more do you need when you have an oil that can cleanse, nourish, purify and protect the skin and hair? Queen of the oils, jojoba is worth every penny. Another advantage of jojoba oil is that it is absorbed quickly by the skin and leaves no residue, so it can be used in all seasons. As jojoba tends not to turn rancid, this preparation will keep for up to 12 months.

2½ tablespoons jojoba oil
5–10 drops essential oil suited to your skin type (optional) (pages 166–70)

– Pour the oils into a bottle and shake well to mix.
– Apply 4–6 drops of the oil to a damp face, leave for 15 minutes, then pat off any excess.

High vibe illuminating moisturiser
For all skin types, especially inflammed and irritated

This intensive rejuvenating moisturiser is great for calming and soothing the skin, while also helping to reduce the appearance of fine lines and wrinkles. The mellow aroma of blue tansy can help to relieve stress and lift one's mood.

4 tablespoons jojoba oil
2 teaspoons rosehip oil
4 drops blue tansy essential oil
4 drops neroli essential oil
2 drops sandalwood essential oil

– Pour the oils into a bottle, shake well to mix.
– Massage 4–6 drops onto a damp face.

GEL MOISTURISER

Gel moisturisers are hydrating, soothing and especially beneficial for oily or sensitive skin. I recommend them for sweltering summer days when the skin tends to become greasy.

Never-an-oily-moment moisturising gel
For oily skin

This soothing and hydrating gel doubles as a great after-sun treatment.

½ teaspoon xanthan gum
5 tablespoons aloe vera juice
1 teaspoon vegetable glycerine
10 drops lavender essential oil

- Using a small mixing wand, slowly mix the gum into the aloe juice until well dissolved and thickened.
- Still blending, add the glycerine and essential oil. Store in the fridge for up to 1 month.

LONG-LIFE EMULSION MOISTURISERS

These emulsions contain only the purest of ingredients and will keep for a long time, especially in the fridge.

Calendula & rose moisturiser
For sensitive skin with thread veins and broken capillaries

This is a lovely, medium-textured, healing and rejuvenating moisturiser for sensitive skin, with or without inflammation. It is also helpful for eczema and wrinkles.

OIL PHASE
7 g plant-derived emulsifying wax
12 ml (¼ fl oz) calendula-infused oil
5 ml (⅛ fl oz) evening primrose oil
5 drops rosemary leaf extract

WATER PHASE

WATER PHASE

75 ml (2½ fl oz) chamomile water
5 ml (⅛ fl oz) vegetable glycerine
12 drops grapefruit seed extract

THIRD PHASE

20 drops rose essential oil (2.5 per cent dilution in jojoba oil)
5 drops German chamomile essential oil (optional)

– Follow the instructions for making an emulsion on page 38.

The immortelle skin moisturiser

For dry, sensitive and mature skin types

One of the most impressive essential oils comes from the resilient yellow-petalled immortelle flower, also aptly known as everlasting, which grows wild in the sandy soils of the Mediterranean coast and possesses incredible powers of longevity: it never wilts. The oil extracted from this plant speeds up cellular turnover and has formidable anti-inflammatory and anti-allergenic properties, making it wonderful for treating eczema and dermatitis.

OIL PHASE

7 g (¼ oz) plant-derived emulsifying wax
2 g (¹⁄₁₆ oz) shea or cocoa butter
15 ml (½ fl oz) calendula-infused oil or sweet almond oil
5 ml (⅛ fl oz) rosehip oil
6 drops rosemary leaf extract

WATER PHASE

75 ml (2½ fl oz) purified water or rosewater
5 ml (⅛ fl oz) vegetable glycerine
15 drops grapefruit seed extract

THIRD PHASE

15 drops neroli essential oil (2.5 per cent dilution in jojoba oil)
5 drops immortelle essential oil

– Follow the instructions for making an emulsion on page 38. Other suggestions: rose and frankincense, combinations for mature skin (pages 166–70).

Lavender & geranium moisturiser with rescue remedy

For all skin types

This is a lovely moisturiser for oily and dehydrated skin wtih vitamin A from carrot oil. Rescue Remedy is available at health food shops and makes an impressive healing addition if your skin is blemished, irritated or angry. Alternatively, you can use an essential oil combination suited to your skin type.

OIL PHASE

6 g (¼ oz) plant-derived emulsifying wax
10 ml (¼ fl oz) jojoba oil
2 ml (⅛ fl oz) carrot-infused oil or rosehip oil
4 drops rosemary leaf extract

WATER PHASE

85 ml (2¾ fl oz) purified water
5 ml (⅛ fl oz) vegetable glycerine
14 drops grapefruit seed extract

THIRD PHASE

10 drops lavender essential oil
10 drops geranium essential oil
6 drops Bach Rescue Remedy (optional)

– Follow the instructions for making an emulsion on page 38.
– Massage into the skin of a night after cleansing and toning.

Exfoliants

Besides a bracing dip in seawater, exfoliating the face with a scrub, peel or cloth is the closest you will get to achieving instant gleaming skin. In fact, there is little more satisfying in the realm of beauty rituals than seeing the skin promptly revitalised. Exfoliating gently lifts layers of dull, dead skin, removes excess sebum and toxins and unblocks pores. This wonderful shedding process also helps promote collagen production, which becomes increasingly important as we mature and our skin's ability to both produce this plumping protein and turn over cells decreases substantially.

While regular exfoliation is widely believed to be one of the keys to retaining and promoting a fresh, dewy, youthful complexion, you must be gentle. Even the slightest irritation or inflammation of the skin can provoke free radical activity, leading to premature ageing of the skin, so gently rub, don't scrub. To ensure your ingredients are ground down as finely as possible, use a coffee grinder, but be sure to invest in separate grinders for your cosmetics and your coffee!

How often you exfoliate depends on the type of peel used, your work and your skin type. Once a week or a fortnight may suit sensitive skin, yet oilier skin may require gentle exfoliation every second day or even daily. Working in greasy kitchens or on dusty building sites will warrant regular, if not daily exfoliation. Winter life spent at home eating rich, fatty foods while huddled up to the heater will leave your skin feeling dry and unbalanced. Before spring, remove the accumulation of toxins and dead skin cells with more regular exfoliation.

Apply and massage exfoliants into a damp face with your fingers. Focus on the areas around your nose, on your forehead and under your lower lip. Avoid the eye area and thread veins.

TYPES OF EXFOLIANT

AHAS occur naturally in fruits, such as citrus, apples and tomatoes and can also be found in fermented dairy products, including yoghurt and kefir. They help to dissolve dead skin cells, clear the pores and reveal a brighter and more radiant complexion.

ENZYMATIC PEELS contain enzymes that help dissolve dead skin cells and clear the pores. Papaya and pineapple contain particularly effective enzymes for this purpose.

FRICTION PEELS dry on the skin and are then gently rubbed off, removing the dead skin cells. These are suited to sensitive, fine and delicate complexions.

GRANULAR SCRUBS lift dead skin cells from the surface of the skin when rubbed. The granules can be made from ground nuts, seeds, grains and pulses. This type of exfoliant is especially beneficial for oilier, congested skin and blocked pores. They are also quite stimulating, benefiting dull, sluggish skin.

MUSLIN OR CHEESECLOTHS are effective exfoliators when a gentle rubbing action is used to remove your preferred cleanser.

WASHING POCHETTES can be made by putting some oatmeal and dried herbs in the middle of muslin (or cheesecloth), tying up the corners and then moistening with lukewarm water before gently washing your face with it. This method works well for sensitive, fragile skin.

SIMPLE SCRUBS

Basic scrub mix
For all skin types

You may substitute any of the ingredients in this scrub mix for other grains and seeds found in your cupboard, as long as they can be ground down very finely. Ground citrus zest, herbs and flowers to suit your skin type also make great additions to this base. For highly sensitive skin, omit the rice flour and double the oatmeal.

    60 g (2 oz/¾ cup) very fine oatmeal
    40 g (1½ oz/⅓ cup) rice flour
    1 tablespoon clay suited to your skin type (page 23)

– Thoroughly combine the ingredients and store in an airtight jar; the mix should last indefinitely if kept dry.
– Put 2 teaspoons of the mixture in a bowl and add enough of a wet ingredient to complement your skin type (honey, yoghurt, milk, egg yolk, fruit, herbal infusions or floral waters – pages 166–70) to form a gritty paste.
– Spread the scrub onto a wet face and massage into the skin using gentle, upward circular motions. Remove with lots of tepid water and a muslin (cheesecloth) wash cloth. Repeat until all the residue is removed. Pat dry.

Here are some exfoliants you can create with or without this basic scrub mix. If you haven't prepared the scrub mix, replace it with a finely ground grain or meal. Apply and remove the scrubs as for the basic scrub mix, unless otherwise stated.

Papaya enzyme scrub
For all skin types

Finely ground adzuki beans have the aroma of freshly cut grass. The Japanese use them to clarify the skin. They grind down to a beautiful and delicate consistency for exfoliation.

    2 teaspoons papaya, mashed
    1 teaspoon adzuki beans, ground

– Combine the ingredients thoroughly.

Brightening strawberry scrub

For oily and combination skin (avoid on sensitive skin)

This fine, fragrant, cleansing and balancing scrub will help clear oily, congested skin and brighten a tired, sallow complexion.

    2 teaspoons basic scrub mix
    1 teaspoon strawberry, mashed
    1 teaspoon natural yoghurt

– Combine the ingredients to form a smooth paste.

Saving grace AHA scrub

For all skin types

By combining a food boasting alpha-hydroxy acids with a grain of some sort in an exfoliant, you get the best of both worlds. The acids in the lemon and milk dissolve impurities, while the grains gently lift them.

    1½ teaspoons basic scrub mix
    1 teaspoon milk of choice
    ½ teaspoon lemon juice

– Combine the ingredients to form a smooth paste.

Seaweed scrub

For all skin types, especially congested or dehydrated

This mineral-rich scrub with malic acid (an AHA found in apples) will help hydrate, smooth and soften the skin.

    1½ teaspoons basic scrub mix
    1½ teaspoons apple juice
    ¼ teaspoon powdered kelp (you can also use spirulina)

– Combine the ingredients to form a smooth paste.

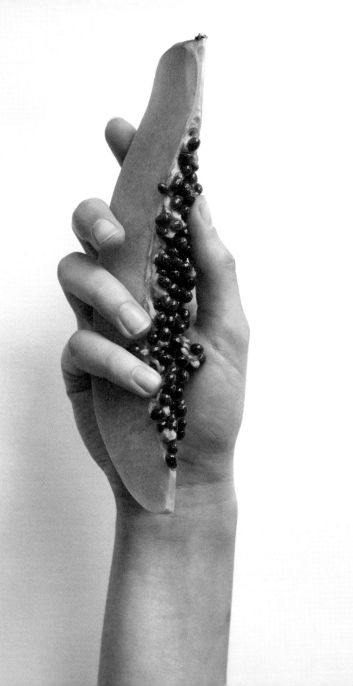

Sweet orange & almond scrub

For all skin types

Bring the rose back into your complexion with this scrub. It is excellent for unplugging blocked pores and smoothing parched and flaky skin.

    2 teaspoons almond meal
    1 teaspoon honey
    1 teaspoon orange juice

– Combine the ingredients thoroughly.

Soothing silk scrub

For mature skin

The perfect antidote to skin chapped by harsh winter weather, this lovely nourishing and emollient scrub leaves the skin feeling soft and glowing. Avocado also works well in place of the banana.

    1½ teaspoons basic scrub mix
    1 teaspoon banana, mashed
    1 teaspoon cream or natural yoghurt
    pinch ground cinnamon (optional)

– Combine the ingredients to form a paste.

LONG-LIFE EXFOLIANTS

These blends will slough off old skin, nourish, cleanse and brighten. They will last 3–6 months in the fridge.

Sandalwood & mandarin face scrub

For sensitive or mature skin

Use this delightful, gentle scrub daily to slough off old skin, nourish, cleanse and brighten the complexion.

   10 drops mandarin essential oil
   5 drops sandalwood essential oil
   70 g (¾ cup) basic scrub mix

– Add the essential oils to the basic scrub mix drop by drop, stirring constantly to avoid clumps.
– Sift then store in an airtight jar.
– To use, mix 1–2 teaspoons with water to form a paste.

Lemon & juniper clay scrub

For oily, combination and congested skin

Juniper is one of the most effective oils for treating congested and blemished skin.

   10 drops lemon essential oil
   10 drops juniper essential oil
   70 g (2½ oz) basic scrub mix

– Add the essential oils to the basic scrub mix drop by drop, stirring constantly to avoid clumps.
– Sift then store in an airtight jar.
– To use, mix 1–2 teaspoons with water to form a paste.

Herbal oats cleansing scrub

For oily, combination and congested skin

This delicious, thick and rich scrub will help clear the pores and prevent blackheads while nourishing the skin. This scrub will keep for up to 3 months in the fridge.

4 tablespoons fine oatmeal

2 tablespoons honey

3 teaspoons distilled witch hazel

1 teaspoon dried and ground peppermint

1 teaspoon dried and ground rosemary

1 teaspoon dried and ground sage

10 drops benzoin essential oil

– Combine the ingredients thoroughly. Store in an airtight jar in the fridge.

Masks

Creating your own wonderful, personalised face mask is akin to cooking a hearty and nourishing casserole without a recipe – rummaging through your cupboard to find anything that will complement the dish. Once you become familiar with the properties of ingredients and what they can do for your skin, you will have the freedom to whip up a mask on the spot. I remember one day a girlfriend came over complaining of tired, greasy and devitalised skin. A couple of very angry spots protruded from her face and she was feeling a little downhearted. I took to the kitchen, apron on, beater and bowl in hand, and swung open the doors to my pantry and fridge to retrieve some remedies. I took a little apple juice mixed with honey, oats, clay, a splashing of wheat germ oil and a drop of lavender essential oil. I cleansed her face, applied a warm compress of water to soften the skin and then slathered on my mask mix from her forehead down to her collarbone. Once the mask was removed, her skin looked calmer and alive, but more importantly, she felt better. Masks not only revitalise the skin but the soul, inspiring time out and leaving you feeling relaxed and pampered. It is believed that the first mask was invented by slave girls in Egypt who were washing their clothes at the Nile's edge. They realised that their feet became soft and pappy after immersion in the mud, and so decided to apply it to their face and hands. Since then, masks have evolved to include a plethora of ingredients that draw dirt, oil and impurities from the skin, soften blackheads, and cleanse, stimulate, soothe, soften, hydrate, balance, nourish, brighten, heal, revitalise and improve the colour, tone and texture of the skin. They can be made from a delicious mix of fresh fruit, veggies, herbs, oils, gels, clays, flours and essential oils.

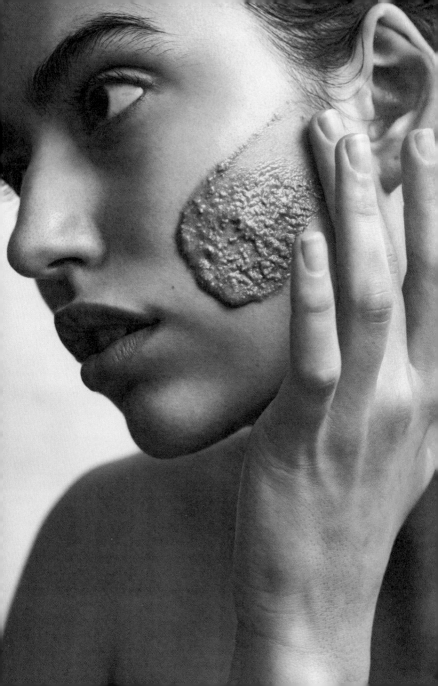

How often you apply a mask depends on the condition of your skin and the type of mask. Normal skin may only need a purifying mask once a week or fortnight, whereas oilier skin will rely on more frequent applications. Mature or dry skin will benefit from a cleansing and nourishing mask at least once a week.

A mask is best applied to a well-cleansed face. For enhanced results, steam your face for 5 minutes before application and frame your face with a hair band to create the perfectly primed canvas. When painting on face masks, skip any broken veins and the delicate skin around the eyes. Instead, coat your eyes with soothing slices of cucumber. Leave masks on for 10–15 minutes. If you have any excess mask, treat your décolletage too. Rinse off with lots of tepid water and a soft cotton cloth and follow with a toner and moisturiser.

TYPES OF MASK

There are two basic types of mask:

DRYING MASKS which dry on the skin, and are predominantly extracting, purifying, stimulating and toning. Argiletz clays, fuller's earth, kaolin, egg and certain gels are common ingredients.

WET MASKS which infuse active ingredients into the skin, hydrate, soothe, calm and heal. They usually stay wet on the skin and are often made from plants, fruit, vegetables, gels, dairy, herbs, egg yolks or honey.

IMPRESSIVE ONE-INGREDIENT FACIALS

AVOCADO is a nourishing and smoothing treat for all skin, especially sensitive, dry and mature.

BREWER'S YEAST stimulates and revives dull, tired skin, and especially benefits oily complexions. Mix with warm water to form a paste and leave on the face for 10 minutes. Avoid on sensitive skin.

SAUERKRAUT JUICE is a naturally-rich in AHAs and detoxifying enzymes, so it's great for helping to refine skin and clear skin breakouts.

CABBAGE is a godsend for treating inflamed, pimpled skin. Dip a couple of cabbage leaves into boiling water to soften them. Once cooled place them over your face for 10 minutes.

CORNFLOUR mixed with a little water makes a soothing mask, brilliant for calming irritated dry skin conditions like eczema.

HONEY spread in a fine layer over your face will help smooth and soften lines, treat skin eruptions, disinfect, cleanse, nourish and tone.

TAHINI a thick, buttery food made from pureed sesame seeds, softens and moisturises dry skin. Spread a fine layer over your face and leave for 10–15 minutes. Rinse off with a cotton cloth and lots of tepid water.

CUSTOMISE YOUR MASK

Basic mask mix
For all skin types

I use this basic mask for a lot of my facials. It is suitable for all skin types and contains healing, nourishing and purifying ingredients. You can add dried and ground herbs and flowers to suit your skin type.

60 g (2 oz/¾ cup) fine oatmeal
50 g (1¾ oz/⅓ cup) clay to suit your skin type (page 23)
2 tablespoons almond meal

– Combine the ingredients and store in a jar in a cool, dark cupboard.
– Mix 1 tablespoon of the basic mix with several ingredients – eggs, yoghurt, milk, dried milk (especially for oily skin), vegetable oils, fruit, vegies, herbs, floral waters, herbal waters or essential oils (1–2 drops per mask) – to make a smooth paste. See pages 166–70 for which ingredients best suit your skin type.
– Note: don't let your mask become so tight that it starts to pull on the skin. Spray regularly with water to soften it. This mask may leave your skin a little red and warm but this should subside within a few minutes. Spray some floral water on your face to cool it down.

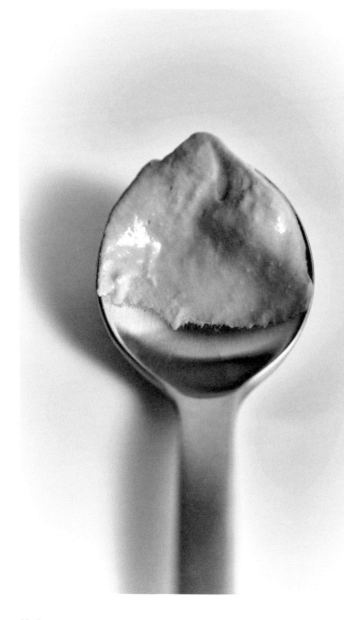

MY FAVOURITE MASK RECIPES

Here are some lovely mask combinations to pep up your complexion.
When it comes to making gel masks with fruit juice, you can either
use fresh juice or grate the fruit and squeeze the juice to produce just
enough for the mask recipe.

Note: if you like your mask more wet, you can add a little more of the
wet ingredients; if you like it drier, add more of the dry ingredients.

Matcha glow mask
For dry, dull skin

Packed with antioxidants from matcha and skin-boosting fatty acids
from coconut oil, this ultra-hydrating mask deeply moisturises skin,
leaving it soft, supple and glowing.

   1 teaspoon matcha green tea powder
   2 teaspoons coconut oil (room temperature and runny)
   ¼ teaspoon honey

– Mix the matcha green tea powder and coconut oil in a bowl until
   well blended.

Fresh herb mask
For all skin types

This delightful mask will cleanse, tone and balance the skin. The live
bacteria in the yoghurt will enhance your skin's health and balance.

   1 teaspoon chopped fresh herbs to suit your skin type (pages 166–70)
   2 teaspoons natural yoghurt
   2 teaspoons basic mask mix

– Pound the herbs using a mortar and pestle and mix with the other
   ingredients.

AHA fruit gel mask

For dehydrated, blotchy or congested skin

A fabulous exfoliating gel mask for unclogging the pores, this will also even up skin tone, improve hydration, and brighten and deep-cleanse the skin. Grape and lemon juice also work well.

> 2 tablespoons apple juice
> 1 tablespoon grapefruit juice
> 1 tablespoon strawberry juice
> 2 teaspoons citrus pectin

– Combine the fruit juices.
– Sprinkle the pectin over the juice mix, then whisk to achieve the desired consistency.

Super power mask

For mature skin

This simple mask is full of antioxidants and AHAs that will soften and revive most complexions. If you wipe this mask off gently with a dry cloth, you'll be amazed at how much dirt it lifts! It works well as a 30-minute mask or left overnight and rinsed off in the morning.

> 2 teaspoons olive oil
> ½ teaspoon lime juice

– Whisk the ingredients to combine until the mixture turns cloudy.

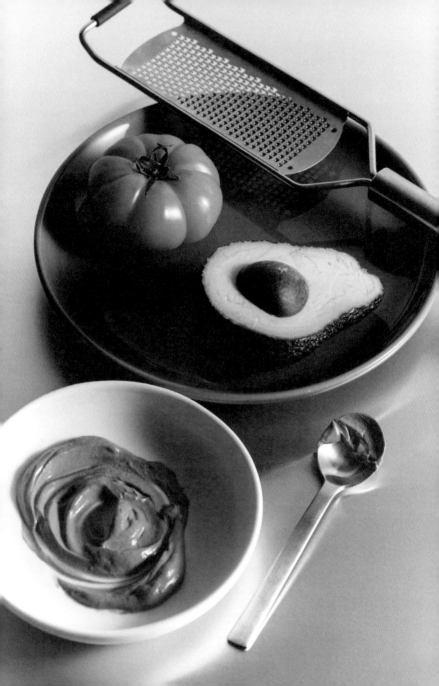

The amazing avocado & tomato mask

For all skin types, except sensitive

This mask lightens and smoothes the complexion beautifully. Tomatoes are full of vitamins A, B and C, AHAs and the potent antioxidant lycopene, while avocado is rich in vitamins, good oils and lecithin.

    2 teaspoons avocado, mashed
    2 teaspoons tomato pulp, grated
    2 teaspoons basic mask mix

– Combine the ingredients thoroughly.

The Korean bath house cucumber milk mask

For all skin types, especially dehydrated and sensitive

When I used to visit the Korean Baths in Sydney, they would lavish a divine mix like this on my face while my body was being scrubbed. This is a delightfully hydrating, soothing and cooling mask.

    2 teaspoons sweet almond oil
    1½ teaspoons honey
    1 tablespoon cucumber, peeled and grated

– Massage the oil into a clean face, spread the honey over the top, then pat the grated cucumber over the honey.

Rose syrup mask

For oily and combination skin

This sweet-scented Ayurvedic mask is very popular among Indian women. It balances and tones oily skin. Lemon juice is ideal for oily, blemish-prone skin because it is antibacterial and contains high levels of vitamin C, which help heal the skin.

    1 tablespoon lemon juice
    1 teaspoon rosewater
    ½ teaspoon honey

– Combine the ingredients thoroughly.

Lavender mud mask

For all skin types, especially dehydrated and congested

Seaplants have been used for centuries for their healing properties by people from many cultures including Chinese, Japanese and Polynesian peoples. Seaplants boast the largest range of minerals of any organism and are used in skincare preparations for their cell-regenerative properties and their ability to attract and retain water. Aloe vera's cosmetic virtues have been extolled since biblical times. Together, the aloe vera juice and the kelp powder make an exceptionally healing, calming, hydrating and regenerative mask that helps reduce the production of excess oil, resulting in a cleaner, clearer complexion with fewer breakouts. If your skin is very dry, add a little avocado or olive oil. This mask is perfect for the advent of spring, when the body needs serious cleansing and detoxification.

    1 tablespoon basic mask mix
    1 teaspoon kelp powder
    3 teaspoons aloe vera juice
    1 drop lavender essential oil

– Thoroughly combine the ingredients.

Pep-me-up papaya mask

For all skin types

Papaya smooths out the skin splendidly without the need to lift a finger! It contains an enzyme called papain, which helps dissolve dead skin cells, thereby pepping up the most tired of complexions. Macadamia nut oil contains palmatoleic acid found in human sebum, making it an excellent oil for mature and dry skin. Sandalwood is remarkably healing, hydrating and balancing, and has the headiest of scents. Spread this mask over your décolletage too. Don't throw the papaya seeds out, as they make a great remedial infusion for a facial steam.

    1 tablespoon mashed papaya flesh
    1 tablespoon basic mask mix
    1 teaspoon macadamia nut oil
    2 drops sandalwood essential oil

– Thoroughly blend the ingredients.

Smoothing honey mask

For dry skin

When your skin needs a simple conditioning treatment, revive it with this lovely old-fashioned and well-known smoothing mix.

1 egg yolk, whipped
1 tablespoon powdered milk (dairy, coconut or oat)
½ teaspoon honey

– Combine the ingredients well.

Pear, sage & green tea cleansing mask

For normal, oily and combination skin

Pears have emollient properties and help moisturise, while green tea is anti-inflammatory and full of antioxidants. Sage is antibacterial, astringent, healing and also very cleansing, making it a wonderful anti-ageing ingredient.

1 tablespoon basic mask mix
1 tablespoon pear, peeled and grated
1 teaspoon strong green tea infusion
1 teaspoon sage infusion

– Thoroughly combine the ingredients.

Supergreens power mask

For congested or tired, dull skin

This nutrient-dense mask is the perfect antidote to revive a tired complexion. Use any greens juice, but this is my favourite combination.

2 tablespoons greens juice:
kale
celery
pineapple
lemon
1 teaspoon citrus pectin, to thicken

– Sprinkle the pectin into the juice and whisk until the mixture forms a gel.
– While your mask settles, drink the rest of your green juice to nourish your gut as well as your skin!

Chamomile, honey & orange blossom gel mask

For sensitive skin

You can use other gelling agents – such as agar-agar and xanthan gum, instead of pectin in this sweetly scented, gentle mask. It will cleanse and soothe sensitive skin.

2 teaspoons strong chamomile infusion
2 teaspoons orange blossom water
1 teaspoon honey
½ teaspoon citrus pectin

- Combine the infusion with the orange water, add the honey and mix thoroughly.
- Sprinkle over the pectin and whisk until the mixture forms a gel.

Aromatic ubtan cinnamon scrub mask

For all skin types

An ubtan is a delicious mask made using grains, herbs and clay mixed with egg. It is pasted on the face and left to set. Then warm milk is spread over the top and the mix is gently rubbed off. This treatment is cleansing, stimulating and excellent for pepping up dull, sluggish skin. You can also use it to 'sand' the body, keeping it soft.

40 g (1½ oz/⅓ cup) basic mask mix
2 tablespoons sandalwood powder
2 teaspoons dried and ground rosehip
1 teaspoon ground cinnamon or nutmeg
1 teaspoon dried and ground orange zest
¼ teaspoon tumeric

- Combine the ingredients thoroughly and store in an airtight jar.
- For normal and combination skin, mix 1 teaspoon with an egg yolk and egg white. For oily skin, mix 1 teaspoon with a whole egg white. For mature or dry skin, mix 1 teaspoon with an egg yolk.
- Apply to the face and leave for 10 minutes.
- Warm a little milk (of your choice), massage into the mask, gently rub the mix off, then rinse.

Manuka honey, carrot & bergamot mask

For acneous, irritated and angry skin

This is an excellent remedial mask for troubled skin. Carrot juice is rich in skin-enhancing compounds, especially the antioxidant beta-carotene. Manuka honey boasts antibacterial properties 20 times stronger than those of tea-tree essential oil. The healing qualities and antidepressive scent of bergamot will help lift dull spirits and calm the complexion.

   1 tablespoon basic mask mix
   2 teaspoons carrot juice
   1 teaspoon Manuka (or ordinary) honey
   1–2 drops bergamot essential oil

– Combine the ingredients until the mixture is smooth.

Coriander mayonnaise mask

For dry and mature skin

A good friend of mine gave me this recipe and it remains one of my favourites. I try to use it once a day for a week every month in winter, to keep my skin well-fed.

   1 egg yolk
   ½ avocado
   ½ bunch fresh coriander
   1 tablespoon natural yoghurt
   1 tablespoon orange juice
   1 teaspoon rosehip oil

– Blend the ingredients until the mixture is smooth.

Miracle spice mask

For oily skin

In India, where a tropical climate means oilier skin and a tendency to collect dust and grime, women herald fenugreek seeds as the miracle spice, with cleansing and rejuvenating properties.

1 tablespoon fenugreek seeds
2 tablespoons natural yoghurt

- Soak the seeds in the yoghurt for an hour, then pummel with a mortar and pestle to make a smooth paste.
- Gently rub the mixture onto the face and neck using circular movements. Leave on for 15 minutes, gently rub off, then rinse with water.

Absolutely fabulous replenishing cream mask

For dry and mature skin

This mask is full of vitamins, fatty acids and antioxidants. Use once a week to revive the skin.

OIL PHASE
9 g (¼ oz) plant-derived emulsifying wax
2 g (¹⁄₁₆ oz) shea or cocoa butter
15 ml (½ fl oz) olive oil
5 ml (⅛ fl oz) rosehip oil
6 drops rosemary leaf extract

WATER PHASE
65 ml (2¼ fl oz) rosewater
5 ml (⅛ fl oz) vegetable glycerine
12 drops grapefruit seed extract

THIRD PHASE
10 drops lavender essential oil
10 drops frankincense essential oil

- Follow the instructions for making an emulsion on page 38.

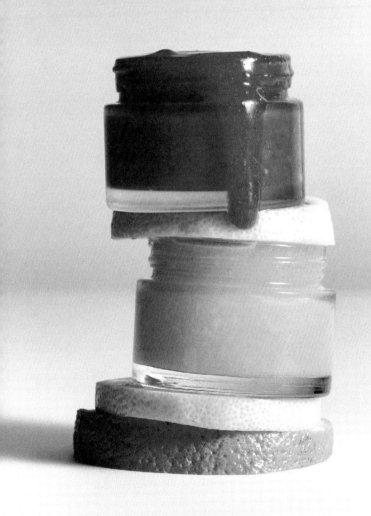

Collagen boost mask

For mature skin and dull, uneven skin tone

When applied topically, vitamin C supports collagen production and helps to even out skin tone, improving the appearance of fine lines, age spots and pigmentation. Papaya and pineapple are not only good sources of vitamin C, but they boost enzymes that help to refine and smooth the complexion.

⅛ teaspoon soluble vitamin C powder (ascorbic acid, preferably with bioflavonoids)

2 teaspoons papaya juice

2 teaspoons pineapple juice

1½ tablespoons basic mask mix

1 drop lemon essential oil (optional)

- Dissolve the vitamin C in the combined papaya and pineapple juices.
- Blend the vitamin mixture with the mask mix to form a smooth paste.
- Add the essential oil and mix well.
- Apply to the face and décolletage, leave for 15 minutes. Warm a little milk, massage into the mask, then rub the mix off. Rinse well.

Hydrating watermelon mask

For dull, dehydrated skin

Watermelon is famous for being ultra-hydrating, but it's also extremely gentle, which makes this mask is suitable for all skin types. This mask will leave your skin looking bright and glowy.

2 tablespoons watermelon juice

1 teaspoon citrus pectin

½ teaspoon runny honey

- Mix the juice and honey together and sprinkle in the citrus pectin and whisk until it forms a gel.

CLAY MASKS

These masks are wonderfully therapeutic and will keep for up to 1 year in the fridge.

Deep-cleansing & balancing clay mask

For oily congested skin

    4 drops orange essential oil
    3 drops palmarosa essential oil
    3 drops sandalwood essential oil
    25 g (1 oz) green clay

– Add the oils to the clay drop by drop and mix thoroughly.
– Sift the mix to remove clumps.
– Combine 1½ teaspoons of the mix with enough water to make a smooth paste.

Calming rose & chamomile mask

For sensitive skin, with or without broken capillaries

This strengthening mask will help calm, tone, decongest and heal the skin while reducing redness and blotchiness.

    6 drops rose essential oil (2.5 per cent dilution in jojoba oil)
    4 drops chamomile essential oil
    25 g (1 oz) pink clay

– Add the oils to the clay drop by drop and mix thoroughly.
– Sift to remove any clumps.
– Combine 1½ teaspoons of the mix with enough water to form a paste.
  Leave on face for five minutes, until almost dry, but don't let dry completely.

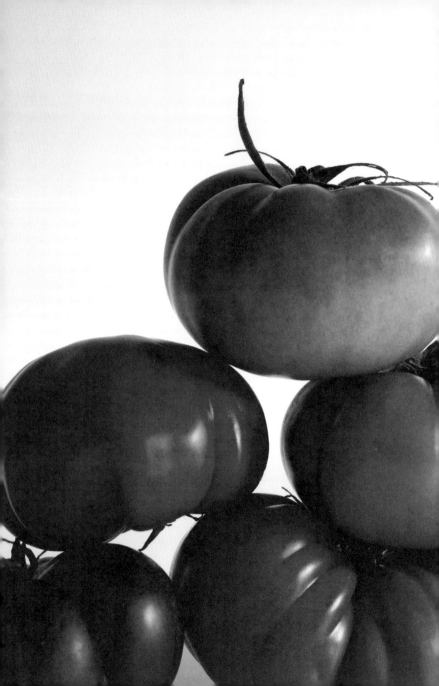

SPOT TREATMENTS

One-ingredient treatments

For acneous skin

To treat blemishes, rub them with nasturtium or calendula (marigold) petals, or coat them with a layer of honey and rinse with warm water after an hour then rub lightly with highly antiseptic garlic cloves.

Bust-my-spot treatment

For acneous skin

This is a very effective zapping treatment for pimples.

    1 tablespoon myrrh tincture
    5 drops lavender essential oil
    5 drops lemon essential oil
    5 drops tea-tree essential oil

– Mix the ingredients thoroughly and apply a small amount to individual blemishes (not the whole face!).

Turmeric paste

For damaged skin

Turmeric is excellent for wound-healing, for bruises and as a decongestant. Mixed with water to form a paste, it also dries out pimples. Leave small spots on for a couple of hours or overnight. Exfoliate the skin gently to remove the stain.

Tomato juice & green clay mask

For acneous skin

Mix about 1 teaspoon of green clay with about ½ teaspoon of tomato juice to form a paste. Tomatoes are high in vitamins A, B and C and AHAs. Together with the extractive properties of green clay, tomato juice makes a formidable mask for spots or acneous patches.

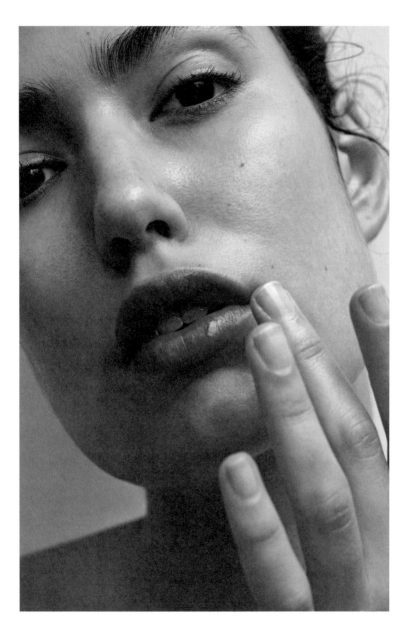

Lips

Lips are hard little workers, contorted many times each day as we express ourselves and, more importantly, exchange warm feelings through a kiss. Without an effective lipid barrier, our lips lose moisture regularly, and their lack of melanin (our body's own protection against sun damage) and sebaceous glands makes them prone to drying out, chapping and developing infections such as cold sores. To sport soft, plump lips, it is vital to wear a natural, protective and vitamin-enriched lip balm daily. To keep moisture trapped, it's important that your lip preparations contain a humectant such as glycerine or honey, or a protective emollient like jojoba.

Most commercial lip preparations are made from petrochemicals, such as petroleum jelly and mineral oils – often alongside other nasty chemicals. The following lip balms and exquisite lip tint are made from natural, health-promoting ingredients like vegetable oils, waxes, extracts, butters and essential oils. You will also find that you don't need to reapply these preparations zillions of times throughout the day. Pucker up and enjoy!

LIP BALMS

Making a lip balm

The natural properties of beeswax soften and protect lips, making it the ideal ingredient for a moisturising lip balm. Your essential oils, in a maximum dilution of 20 drops for every 100 g (3½ oz) of balm, should be non-toxic and should not photosensitise the skin. Here is a basic balm-making method to use with the recipes that follow.

– Melt the beeswax and/or cocoa butter and/or shea butter in a bain-marie.
– Add the vegetable oil and/or honey, keeping the mixture over heat.
– Using a small mixing wand, beat well to blend the ingredients.
– Remove from heat and, once the mixture begins to cool, stir in any essential oils.
– Pour into small jars, lipstick moulds or pretty tin pillboxes.
– For a lovely shine, use a lip brush to apply.

Basic healing lip balm

10 ml (¼ fl oz) vitamin E oil (tocopherol)
50 ml (1¾ fl oz) jojoba oil
10 g (¼ oz) beeswax

– Mix the vitamin E into the jojoba oil then follow the instructions for making a lip balm above.

Mandarin & anise lip gloss

Anise has a delicious aroma, reminiscent of licorice. It has reputed aphrodisiac powers and helps allay frazzled nerves. Mandarin will also help calm the mind.

12 g (½ oz) beeswax
8 g (¼ oz) cocoa butter
50 ml (1¾ fl oz) calendula-infused oil
½ teaspoon honey
9 drops mandarin essential oil
6 drops anise essential oil

– Follow the instructions for making a lip balm above.

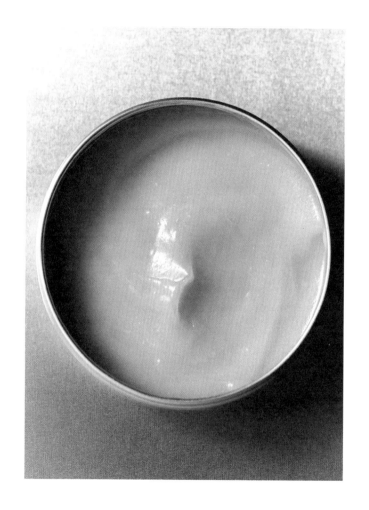

Lips

Lime & sandalwood healing lip balm

Shea butter is a wonderful emollient that softens and helps repair the skin on the lips.

15 g (½ oz) beeswax
5 g (⅛ oz) shea butter
50 ml (1¾ fl oz) jojoba oil
5 ml (⅛ fl oz) calendula-infused oil
8 drops lime essential oil
7 drops sandalwood essential oil

– Follow the instructions for making a lip balm on page 98.

LIP TINT

Beetroot & orange lip & cheek tint

Layer the healing lip balm on top of this rosy tint for shiny pink lips.

2 teaspoons beetroot powder or crystals
3 teaspoons vodka
¼ teaspoon vegetable glycerine
3 drops sweet orange essential oil

– Dissolve the beetroot powder in the vodka.
– Add the glycerine and oil, mixing well.
– Apply with a brush. Store in a bottle for up to 3 months in the fridge.

LIP TREATMENTS

EXFOLIATION To keep your lips in good shape, exfoliate regularly and gently with a soft children's toothbrush or damp face washer.

HONEY To help smooth the lips, layer resinous honey over them and leave for 15 minutes or longer.

VITAMIN E A few drops rubbed into the lips and left overnight make a wonderful nourishing and healing treatment.

Cold sore healing preparation

A potent essential oil blend to help relieve cold sores.

    5 drops geranium essential oil
    5 drops lavender essential oil
    5 drops tea-tree essential oil
    1 tablespoon myrrh tincture

– Add the essential oils to the tincture, bottle and shake well to mix.
– Apply the preparation sparingly to the cold sore throughout the day.

Plumping lip scrub

A delicious lip scrub to help slough off flaky skin. Peppermint oil is stimulating and will help bring blood flow to your lips for a smoother, plumper pout.

    2 tablespoons finely ground sugar
    2 teaspoons coconut oil
    2 teaspoons almond oil
    2 drops peppermint oil

– Combine all ingredients together until well mixed.
– Gently massage ½–1 teaspoon of the scrub to your lips.
– Wash off with a warm cloth.

Eyes

The delicate skin that cradles the eyes is stretched, twisted and scrunched countless times a day as we laugh, weep, squint at bright lights, wince at dusty city air, blink to keep our eyes moist and, as the evening approaches, struggle to keep our peepers open. Because this area has fewer oil glands than the rest of the face, it is far more prone to lines and wrinkles.

Regular application of eye creams, gels and oils will help prevent, reduce and smooth out cracks and crevices and keep the skin plump and hydrated. Rich and heavy creams will only drag the skin down in that area, exacerbating already existing lines and creating new ones, so opt for feather-light creams and apply them gently around the orbital bone, using the gentle touch of your middle finger.

Try not to be too critical of those fine character lines – the eyes can be the windows to our soul and a few laughter lines surrounding them are an endearing and welcoming feature.

When shopping for eye creams, avoid formulas that contain alcohol as they may temporarily tighten the area but are harsh and can irritate the skin. Certain herbs can also be used to ameliorate other common problems, such as dark circles and bags.

Eyebright

As its name indicates, the herb eyebright has long been used to add a special shine to the eyes. Mix 20 drops of tincture of eyebright into a glass of chilled distilled water and apply morning and night to closed eyes using cotton makeup pads or a cloth.

PUFFINESS & DARK CIRCLES

Finger treatment

Puffiness around the eyes can be reduced by gently patting the bone around the eye with a finger (middle is best).

The magic spoon treatment

One of my favourite tricks is to put stainless steel spoons in the freezer for 10 minutes and then place them over my eyes for a few minutes. This is a fabulous way of reducing puffiness before going out or after a late night.

Potato treatment

To help lighten the appearance of dark circles and tighten skin, grate a raw potato, wrap it in muslin (cheesecloth) and apply to eyelids for 15–20 minutes. Gently wash off any residue and then apply a light eye cream or jojoba oil.

FRESH FOOD REMEDIES

Here are some effective ways to combat tired, puffy eyes and dark circles using fresh ingredients.

BUTTERMILK tones under the eyes, helping restore the acid mantle.

CUCUMBER tones up the skin around the eyes and cools and soothes inflamed eyes. Use a slice of peeled cucumber as an eye pad.

TEAS Place wet, chilled tea bags or cotton makeup pads, soaked in tea over closed eyes. This will soothe irritated, gritty and puffy eyes. Black, calendula, chamomile, fennel, green, parsley, red clover and rosehip teas all work well.

FRESH FIG on closed eyes will reduce puffiness.

FRESH COLD MILK Soak cotton makeup pads in milk and place over closed eyes for 10 minutes.

WITCH HAZEL Chill and apply to closed eyes using cotton makeup pads.

EYE SOOTHERS

Regenerative eye oil
For all skin types

Rosehip oil is very popular in regenerative skincare. It is extracted from the fruit of a rose bush that grows wild in the southern Andes and is extremely beneficial in tissue regeneration for burns, facial wrinkles and scars, due to its high concentration of fatty acids. Rosehip oil makes an excellent night oil for mature skin, and also those with oily skin, because of its high content of both fatty acids and trans-retinoic acid. I often add a couple of drops of immortelle essential oil to this mix, as it seems to help diminish puffiness around the eyes. This oil will keep for up to 1 year.

2 tablespoons jojoba oil
2 teaspoons rosehip oil
5 drops immortelle essential oil (optional)

- Pour or drop the oils into a bottle and shake well to combine.
- Moisten the skin around and under the eye. Pat on a few drops of the oil using the middle finger of your chosen hand. Keep patting gently until most of the oil is absorbed. Leave for 20 minutes and then blot off any surplus oil.

Soothing eye cream

For all skin types

This is a light moisturising cream for around the eyes. Rose and carrot seed oil both improve skin tone and elasticity and help the appearance of wrinkles.

OIL PHASE

7 g (¼ oz) plant-derived emulsifying wax
10 ml (¼ fl oz) apricot kernel oil
5 ml (⅛ fl oz) rosehip oil
4 drops rosemary leaf extract

WATER PHASE

70 ml (2¼ fl oz) rosewater
5 ml (2½ fl oz) vegetable glycerine
15 drops grapefruit seed extract

THIRD PHASE

5 drops carrot seed essential oil
10 drops rose essential oil (2.5 per cent dilution in jojoba oil)

– Follow the instructions for making an emulsion on page 38.

EYE MASK

Soothing cucumber milk mask

This is a lovely, gentle, soothing and slightly toning eye mask.

2 teaspoons cucumber, peeled and grated
1 tablespoon powdered milk (powdered coconut or oat milk)
1 teaspoon honey

– Combine the ingredients to form a paste.
– Apply over and around closed eyes. Leave for about 10 minutes then rinse with cool water and follow with the regenerative eye oil (opposite).

Body

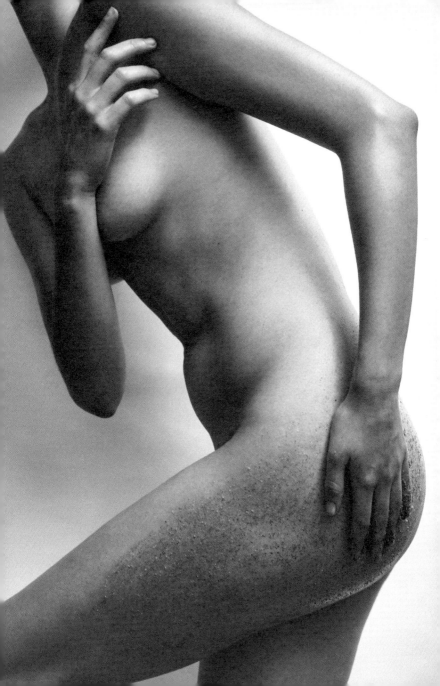

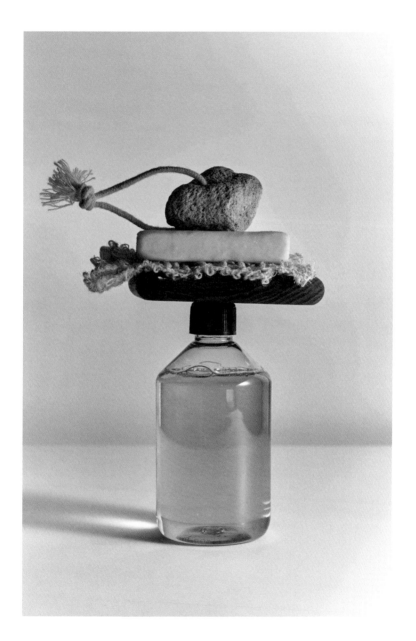

All over

Ruddy décolletages and coarse, parched body skin are often caused by a lack of moisture, a poor diet and not enough protection from the sun's rays. Mediterranean cultures have always recognised the importance of sustaining the body with nourishing foods that can counteract the damaging effects of a hot climate. In Greece, pomegranate, one of the most potent anti-ageing fruits, is still revered for its protective qualities. It contains three times the antioxidants of green tea. When eaten or applied topically, this bejewelled fruit helps ravage free radicals, preventing them from wreaking havoc in the body and on the skin. A well-known recipe in Greece is a delicious body butter of macerated pomegranate, beeswax and olive oil. Many Greek people apply this rich mixture all over their bodies each day to ensure healthy, gleaming skin.

If your temple is looking a little broken or weathered, some love, attention and fresh food therapy will help rebuild its beautiful and unique structure. Remember, a wholesome diet and lots of exercise and relaxation are your body's supporting pillars. Shun harsh chemical cleansers that strip the skin, and lavish organic foods, essential oils and nutritious ingredients on your precious self to feed, nurture and revitalise from top to toe.

BODY CLEANSERS

Make-me-over body cleanser
For all skin types

This gentle foaming cleanser will leave your body fragrant, soft and squeaky clean. It will last up to 6 months when stored in a cool place, away from direct sunlight. For extra healing and cleansing properties, add 2 teaspoons of a clay that suits your skin type (see page 23).

    4 tablespoons liquid Castile soap
    2 teaspoons sweet almond oil
    20 drops essential oil (optional)

– Pour or drop the ingredients into a bottle and shake well to combine. Shake well before each use.

Depending on your mood, try one of these essential oil combinations: relaxing – 8 drops bergamot, 8 lavender, 6 chamomile; refreshing – 8 drops orange, 6 grapefruit, 6 lime; and antiseptic – 8 drops geranium, 8 lavender, 6 tea-tree.

BODY BUFFING

Buffing the body with a natural-bristle brush or natural homemade body scrub is one of the quickest ways to achieve healthy, lustrous skin. As the skin on the body is much tougher than on the face, you can scrub firmly, using bigger, sharper granules, like sugar and salt. Blemishes on the body, like those on the face, can reflect a deficiency in the diet or toxicity. So while following these delicious recipes will be of assistance, it's also important to look at your lifestyle.

Dry skin body brushing
For all skin types

This very old and revered technique not only whisks away built-up dead skin cells, but kickstarts the lymphatic system, helping to eliminate a generous portion of the body's waste. It helps to stimulate and tone the skin. I always feel like I've been for a good half-hour walk after brushing for a few minutes.

Stand bare in a comfortable space and stretch your whole body from the tips of your toes to the top of your head to awaken the senses. Starting at the feet, make long sweeping strokes over the front and backs of the legs. Brush over the bottom and up to the mid-back. Brush your hands, arms, across the shoulders, up the neck, down the chest (skipping the nipples!) and down to the tummy. Using circular motions, brush the abdomen in a clockwise direction. Remember: always work towards the heart and then stroke downward, pushing toxins toward the colon. Follow with a warm shower, finished with 10 seconds of cold water. Avoid brushing too vigorously or you may scratch the skin. If the skin on your body is very sensitive, invest in a soft-bristled brush.

BODY SCRUBS

Body scrubs feel wonderful and can help to relieve itchy, flaking skin. Salt and sugar are both perfect bases to which to add vegetable oils, infused oils, herbs and essential oils, as they do not create a big sodden mess like grains. Apply all scrubs to a damp body, massage into the skin, then rinse well.

Fresh ginger scrub
For cellulite

The Japanese have used this scrub for centuries. Mix 2 teaspoons of grated ginger with 2 tablespoons of sea salt and rub into cellulite to help decongest fatty deposits and improve circulation.

Coconut & cocoa body scrub

For all skin types

Coffee stimulates and dispels congestion, while cocoa powder is a wonderful way to promote cell renewal and skin healing.

    460 g (1 lb/2 cups) coconut or raw sugar
    125 ml (4 fl oz/½ cup) sweet almond oil
    125 ml (4 fl oz/½ cup) coconut oil (room temperature)
    2 tablespoons cocoa powder
    2 tablespoons ground coffee
    2 teaspoons vanilla extract

– Mix all ingredients thoroughly and put into an airtight jar. This will keep for up to 6 months.

Celtic salt body scrub

For all skin types, except very sensitive

This simple salt scrub polishes to perfection. Warning: oily preparations can make the shower recess very slippery!

    240 g (8½ oz /1 cup) celtic or finely granulated sea salt
    20–40 drops essential oil of your choice (optional; see the oil combinations on page 124 for ideas)
    125 ml (4 fl oz/½ cup) sweet almond or other cold-pressed vegetable oil

– Pour the salt into an airtight preserving jar.
– Add the essential oils to the base oil drop by drop and blend.
– Pour the oil mixture into the salt. Seal the jar and shake well. This mixture will keep for up to 6 months.

Poppyseed & orange body scrub

For all skin types

This zesty scented orange scrub helps to revitalise the body.

    210 g (7½ fl oz/1 cup) sugar
    85 g (3 oz/½ cup) apricot kernel oil or sweet almond oil
    2 tablespoons poppyseeds
    30 drops sweet orange essential oil

– Use the same method as for Coconut & cocoa body scrub (above).

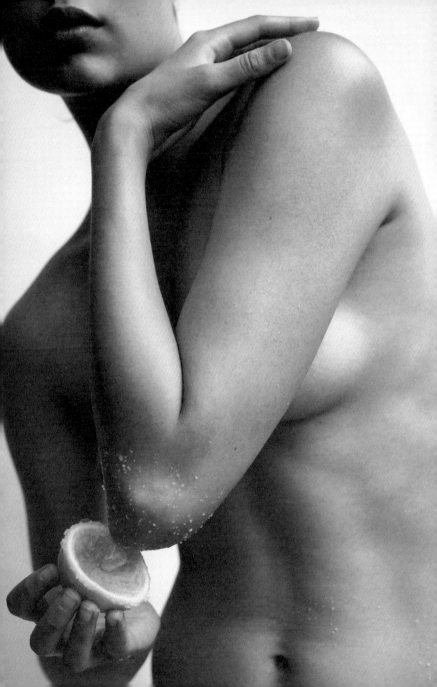

Pink tangerine, rosewood & lavender scrub

For sensitive skin

This also makes a balancing body scrub that you can leave on as a mask for 15 minutes.

10 drops lavender essential oil
10 drops tangerine essential oil
10 drops rosewood essential oil
2 tablespoons pink clay
120 g (4½ oz/1¼ cups) fine oatmeal
2 teaspoons chamomile flowers, dried and finely ground

– Drop the oils into the clay.
– Sift out any wet clumps.
– Add the oatmeal and the chamomile flowers. Store in an airtight container.
– Combine 3 tablespoons of the mix with enough water or milk to form a paste.

Green clay scrub with salt, rice, bergamot, lavender & ylang-ylang

For oily or blemished skin

Without the salt, this makes a clarifying body mask for oily skin.

10 drops bergamot essential oil
10 drops lavender essential oil
6 drops ylang-ylang essential oil
2 tablespoons green clay
100 g (3½ oz/¾ cup) rice flour
3 tablespoons sea salt

– Drop the oils into the clay.
– Sift out any wet clumps.
– Add the rice flour and the sea salt. Store in an airtight container.
– Combine 3 tablespoons of the mix with enough water or milk to form a paste.

BODY MASKS

When planning to dress your body in a mask, make sure you have enough time, space, privacy, towels and running water before you start – the simplest tasks can be difficult to negotiate when you're smothered in a thick layer of goo.

Olive oil antioxidant mask

For all skin types, except very oily

Olive oil is full of antioxidants and makes a wonderfully nourishing and strengthening skin treatment. Slather a thoroughly cleansed body with olive oil, then pop on some old cotton clothes for 1 hour. Take the clothes off and your body will be soft and supple. You don't need to wash off the oil; by the time it has been absorbed by both your clothes and skin there shouldn't be any left.

Sundari body mask with avocado & rose geranium

Sundari means 'beautiful woman' in Sanskrit. Make fresh as needed.

 2 tablespoons pink clay
 2 tablespoons papaya, fleshed, mashed
 1 teaspoon avocado oil
 5 drops rose geranium essential oil (optional)

– Combine all the ingredients to form a paste.
– Spread over a clean, damp body, leave for 10–15 minutes, then rinse.

White rice miso & honey body paste

White rice shiro miso mixed with honey makes a rich and delicious body paste. Miso is full of skin-smoothing amino acids. Extend this to your face for a nourishing treat.

 2 tablespoons honey
 1 teaspoon vanilla extract
 1 tablespoon white rice shiro miso

– Combine the ingredients to form a smooth paste.
– Spread over a clean, damp body, leave for 10–15 minutes, then rinse well.

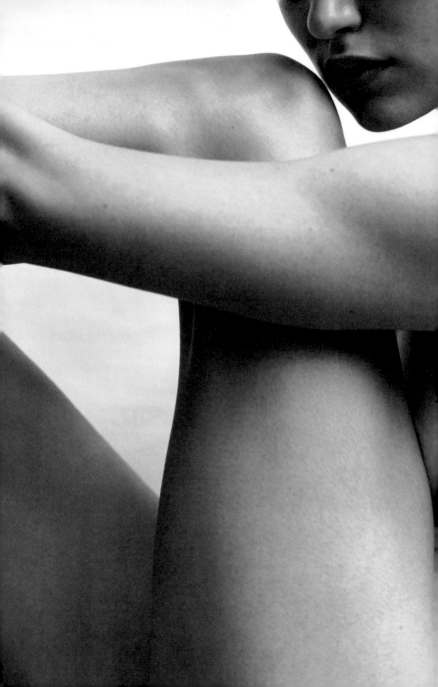

Papaya polishing mask
For all skin types

To dissolve dead skin cells and soften the skin, rub the insides of a papaya skin all over a clean, damp body. Leave for 20 minutes then rinse off.

Ayurvedic bridal body mask
For all skin types

This wonderful mask recipe was shared with me by a friend who pioneered Ayurvedic treatments in Australia. Traditionally used by Indian brides, the mask is prepared 10 days before the wedding and applied every day until the ceremony for soft, clear, fragrant skin.

4 tablespoons finely ground wheat germ
2 tablespoons ground almond meal
1 tablespoon dried and ground orange peel
1 tablespoon dried and ground lemon peel
1 tablespoon ground thyme
½ tablespoon ground turmeric
pinch salt
2 drops rose or jasmine essential oil

- Combine the dry ingredients thoroughly.
- Add the essential oil drop by drop and mix well.
- Store in an airtight jar.
- Combine 3–4 tablespoons of the mix with enough sweet almond oil to form a smooth paste, spread over a clean, damp body and leave for 20 minutes. Firmly rub off the dried mask and rinse well.

BODY MOISTURISERS

Keep the body nourished and supple with these wonderful moisturising preparations.

Frankincense, bergamot & lime smoothing cream
For all skin types

This uplifting, soothing, hydrating and non-greasy lotion is easily absorbed by thirsty skin.

OIL PHASE

9 g (¼ oz) plant-derived emulsifying wax

2 g ($\frac{1}{16}$ oz) cocoa butter

20 ml (¾ fl oz) sweet almond oil

6 drops rosemary leaf extract

WATER PHASE

170 ml (5½ fl oz) purified water, floral water or aloe vera juice

8 ml vegetable glycerine

34 drops grapefruit seed extract

THIRD PHASE

18 drops bergamot essential oil

18 drops lime essential oil

12 drops frankincense essential oil

– Follow the instructions for making an emulsion on page 38.

Flower power body balm

For mature, dry skin

Ylang-ylang, patchouli and rose make a divinely scented mix. Ylang-ylang has a balancing effect on skin, making it ideal for all skin types, while its jasmine-like, heady fragrance is also a renowned aphrodisiac. Patchouli and rose are also famed for inspiring good loving.

OIL PHASE

16 g (½ oz) plant-derived emulsifying wax

10 g (¼ oz) cocoa butter

40 ml (1¼ fl oz) sweet almond oil

5 ml (⅛ fl oz) evening primrose oil

12 drops rosemary leaf extract

WATER PHASE

120 ml (4 fl oz) rosewater

8 ml (¼ fl oz) vegetable glycerine

25 drops grapefruit seed extract

THIRD PHASE

15 drops patchouli essential oil

15 drops palmarosa essential oil

10 drops neroli essential oil (2.5 per cent dilution in jojoba oil)

10 drops ylang-ylang essential oil

– Follow the instructions for making an emulsion on page 38.

BODY POWDER

Body powders absorb perspiration and moisture from the skin, making them ideal for balmier weather, when clothes tend to rub against sweaty skin and cause chafing and irritation. Body powders can also be dusted over the body after a shower or bath to help speed up drying time and to lightly scent the body. Powders of arrowroot, cornflour (cornstarch), orris root flour, potato flour, rice flour and white clay can be used alone or in combination.

Basic dusting powder
For all skin types

To make a deodorising powder for under the arms, add ¼ cup of bicarbonate of soda (baking soda) to this combination. Orris root comes from the Florentine iris and boasts a beautiful delicate scent, reminiscent of violets.

> 50 g (1¾ oz) white clay powder
> 70 g (2½ oz) fine cornflour (cornstarch) or orris root powder
> 20 drops essential oil of your choice

– Combine the dry ingredients in a completely dry blender.
– Add the essential oil drop by drop and blend until mixed thoroughly.
– Sift to remove any lumps. Decant the powder into a salt or parmesan shaker for easy dusting onto the body, or use a powder puff to apply.

Here are some deliciously fragrant essential oil combinations for your powder:

SENSUAL AND SPICY – 10 drops orange, 8 sandalwood, 2 cinnamon

SOFT LAVENDER – 8 drops bergamot, 6 lavender, 6 natural vanilla essence

EXOTIC FLORAL – 8 drops rose, 7 jasmine, 5 ylang-ylang

UPLIFTING – 10 drops lavender, 6 geranium, 4 nutmeg

DEODORISING – 9 drops lemon, 6 patchouli, 4 myrrh

CITRUS – 12 drops grapefruit, 6 bergamot, 4 orange

FRESH SPRING – 6 drops palmarosa, 4 rosewood, 2 geranium.

DEODORANTS

The pheromones released in our sweat may influence both who we attract and who we are attracted to, and yet we so often quash this natural body chemistry with the use of deodorants. Natural deodorants do not prevent perspiration, which is important, because sweating out unwanted toxins is necessary for healthy body function. Instead, they mask the odour and may inhibit the growth of bacteria.

Sage has been used for hundreds of years to control body odour and lovage was a favourite deodorant among ancient herbalists. Other effective deodorising herbs are basil, calendula, eucalyptus, lavender, lemongrass, mint, rosemary, sage, spearmint, tea-tree, thyme, yarrow, or any other appealing pungent herb. For a deodorant, make a 50 per cent dilution in water of a herbal vinegar made with a combination of these herbs. All green leafy vegetables are high in chlorophyll and can be rubbed into the armpits to reduce perspiration odour. If your odour is pungent, try rubbing some watercress or parsley under your arms before spritzing with the following spray. Bicarbonate of soda (baking soda) is also very effective.

Patchouli and lime deodorant spray
For all skin types

Patchouli essential oil has been used for centuries to mask body odour and cypress is renowned for quashing wetness. This spray has a sweet, heady and sensual aroma you'll love.

   3 tablespoons distilled witch hazel
   2 tablespoons vodka
   2 teaspoons glycerine
   15 drops bergamot essential oil
   15 drops citrus seed extract
   10 drops lime essential oil
   10 drops patchouli essential oil
   5 drops cypress essential oil

– Combine the ingredients and store in a spray bottle in the fridge
  for up to 1 year.

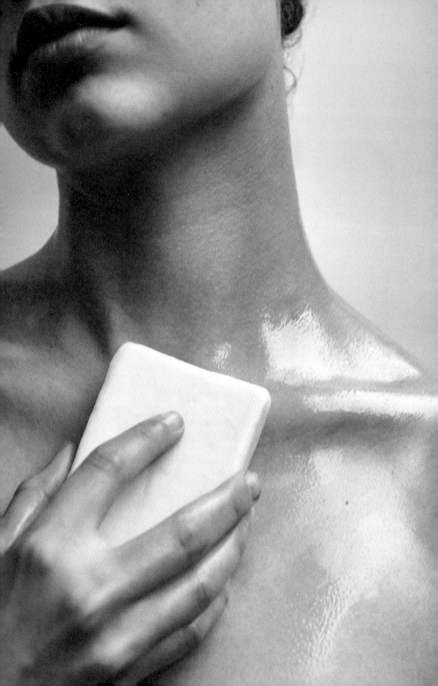

BODY OILS

A body massage is one of life's most pleasurable experiences – we all need to be touched and nurtured by other human beings. A massage also has many health benefits: it stimulates the circulatory and lymphatic systems, increasing the elimination of toxins and improving muscle and skin tone; and it arouses and soothes the nervous system, resulting in a feeling of wellbeing and relaxation.

Vegetable oils are nourishing and can be used alone or with essential oils. They are the perfect vehicle for carrying essential oils deep into the skin and throughout the whole body. This penetration takes around 20 minutes.

To prevent deterioration of your oil, add 10 per cent vitamin E oil. Recommended massage base oils are sweet almond, apricot kernel, sunflower, safflower, soybean, olive and jojoba.

Herbal infused oils

Herbal infused oils make wonderfully therapeutic massage oils. Choose herbs to suit your skin type (pages 166–70) and follow the instructions for making an infused oil on page 33.

Orange blossom body spray

This is a delightfully fragrant and uplifting orange-scented body spray. Neroli oil is extracted from the white blossoms of the bitter orange tree, petitgrain from the leaves of the bitter orange tree and sweet orange from the peel of the orange.

    10 drops neroli essential oil
    10 drops petitgrain essential oil
    10 drops sweet orange essential oil
    2 tablespoons vodka
    3 tablespoons orange blossom water

- Stir the essential oils into the vodka, then mix with the orange blossom water.
- Pour into a spray bottle. Shake well before each use.

Aromatherapy massage oils

For a typical aromatherapy massage, mix 15–25 drops of essential oil with 3 tablespoons of carrier oil. Here are some suggestions:

ENERGISING – 10 drops grapefruit, 8 bergamot, 4 peppermint

DETOXIFYING AND STIMULATING (good for cellulite) – 10 drops grapefruit, 8 lemon, 6 juniper

TONING – 6 drops cypress, 6 lemon, 6 patchouli, 6 rose

RELAXING – 10 drops sandalwood, 8 neroli, 8 rose

FOR LOVERS – 10 drops orange, 6 patchouli, 4 cinnamon, 4 ylang-ylang

FOR STRETCH MARKS – 5 drops lavender, 5 mandarin.

Cocoa massage bars with mandarin, lime & nutmeg

Use this as a massage bar, or cut off a sliver and pop it in your bath. Massage it into cuticles, heels and elbows.

140 g (5 oz) cocoa butter
10 g (¼ oz) beeswax
2 tablespoons coconut oil
30 drops lime essential oil
30 drops mandarin essential oil
8 drops nutmeg essential oil

– Melt the cocoa butter, beeswax and coconut oil in a bain-marie and mix well.
– Remove from the heat for a few minutes then add the essential oils.
– Pour into moulds then refrigerate to harden. Store in the fridge.

Jasmine-infused body gloss

The warm, heady perfume of jasmine is synonymous with love and sex; it is mentioned in the *Kamasutra* as a fragrance that penetrates the five senses. It increases the beta waves in the brain, making you more aware of everything around you.

At the end of winter and beginning of spring, when jasmine is starting to bloom, I put jasmine petals in a bottle of apricot kernel oil and infuse them for 10 days (page 33). Sometimes I throw dried mandarin peel into the mix to give a little citrus flavour to this floral oil. It makes a lovely skin gloss for balmy evenings out. To enhance the fragrance, add a few drops of jasmine and mandarin essential oils. Ylang-ylang, neroli, sweet orange, patchouli and sandalwood also work well.

Spice-scented spice body oil

This lovely woody, aromatic body oil can be massaged onto limbs or used as a bath oil.

2 whole cloves
1 cinnamon stick
1 large bay leaf, crushed
1 vanilla pod, split and cut into pieces
125 ml (4 fl oz/½ cup) jojoba oil or sweet apricot kernel oil
10 drops patchouli essential oil
30 drops sweet orange essential oil (optional)

- Infuse the herbs and spices in the jojoba oil for 2 weeks (see page 33).
- Strain through coffee filter paper.
- Add the patchouli oil and the sweet orange oil if using.
- Leave to mellow for 2 weeks before use.

INSECT REPELLENT

Don't bug me

I have an aversion to most commercial insect repellents, which
usually contain a whole host of dubious synthetic chemicals.
Certain essential oils are extremely good at repelling little bugs;
I like to add them to a balmy base that will roll onto the skin easily.
If you prefer a spray, use the Patchouli and lime deodorant spray base
(page 121) to carry the essential oils below. Citronella and lemon are
also impressive insect repellents. Damp green tea leaves rubbed on
insect bites will help relieve itching, while fresh basil leaves or slices
of onion will also relieve stinging.

15 g (½ oz) beeswax
10 g (¼ oz) cocoa butter
3½ tablespoons sweet almond oil
20 drops geranium essential oil
20 drops lavender essential oil
15 drops lemongrass essential oil

– Melt the beeswax and cocoa butter in a bain-marie, mixing well to combine.
– Remove from heat for a few minutes, then add the essential oils.
– Pour into a mould then allow to solidify at room temperature.
  Store in the fridge.

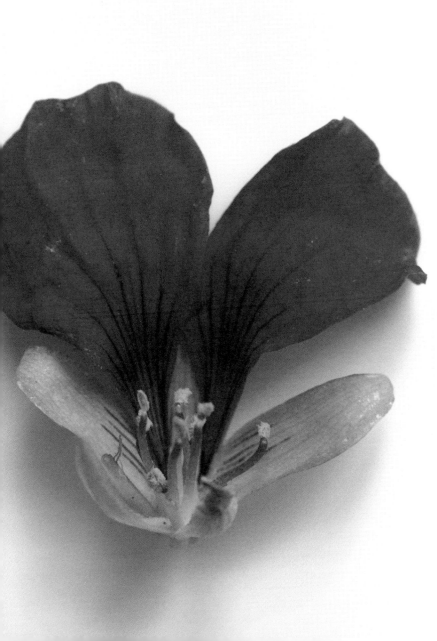

Neck

The neck is one of the first places to show signs of ageing. Engage in regular neck exercises and facial yoga to firm up those defiant muscles, and apply a nourishing and firming mask weekly. Extend your facial toners, exfoliants and moisturisers to your neck, using light, upward, feathery strokes.

HERBAL NECK TONERS

Stimulate and firm the dry and lined areas of the neck with herbal infusions that have astringent properties. Suitable herbs are horsetail, lime flower, nettle, peppermint, sage or thyme.

Replenishing neck and breast oil

For all skin types

This lovely light oil will help keep the neck toned and moisturised.

    2 tablespoons apricot kernel oil
    1 tablespoon jojoba oil
    2 tablespoons rosehip oil
    8 drops neroli essential oil (2.5 per cent dilution in jojoba oil)
    6 drops lavender essential oil
    4 drops frankincense essential oil

- Pour or drop the oils into a bottle and shake to combine.
- Massage into the neck using upward, circular motions.

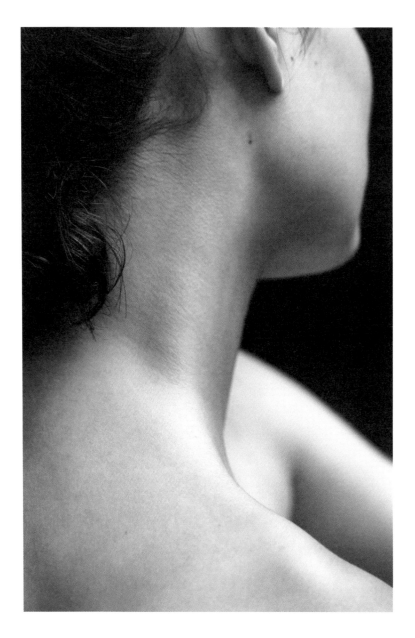

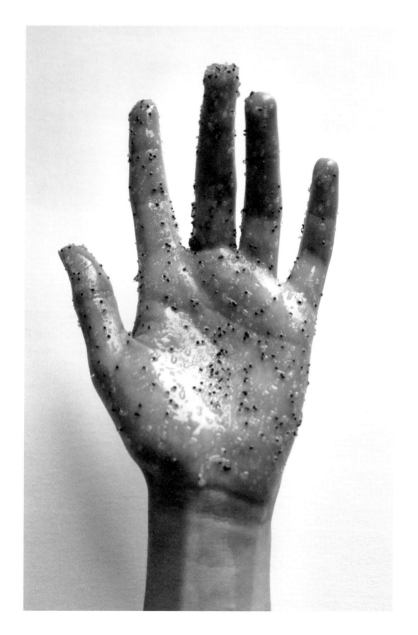

Hands

We anoint our faces and necks with the finest concoctions to help keep them soft and supple, but neglect to pamper our diligent and tactile hands, which are constantly on display to the world. My grandmother would say that hands give away your age far quicker than the face. The skin on the hands lacks oil glands, and so is very prone to dryness and premature ageing. Add years of washing in solvents, sun exposure and general wear and tear, and they can become more susceptible to skin conditions such as dermatitis. To protect them and keep them soft and smooth, slip on cotton gloves under your rubber set when washing up to prevent perspiration and irritation. When gardening, opt for reinforced fabric gloves. Avoid using harsh soaps and apply a homemade hand cream after washing to replace lost moisture.

HAND CLEANSERS & SCRUBS

Soft as silk hand cleanser
For all skin types

Keep a small jar of coarse oatmeal near the sink. Spoon 1 teaspoon into the palm of your hand, mix with water and rub your hands together thoroughly to cleanse. Add 5 drops of lavender oil to the jar for a fragrant and antiseptic cleanse.

Refreshing grapefruit soap hand wash
For all skin types

This is a lovely refreshing and antiseptic foaming cleanser.

  2½ tablespoons liquid Castile soap
  1 teaspoon olive oil
  10 drops grapefruit essential oil

− Pour or drop the ingredients into a bottle and shake well to combine.

Sugar & lime hand scrub
For all skin types

This lovely weekly treat for dry, flaky, dull and mottled hands will smooth and brighten. It smells sweetly of freshly peeled lime zest.

  4 tablespoons granulated raw sugar
  2 tablespoons sweet almond oil
  10 drops distilled lime essential oil

− Combine the ingredients thoroughly and store in an airtight jar.
− Massage 1 teaspoon of the mixture into dampened hands, then rinse.

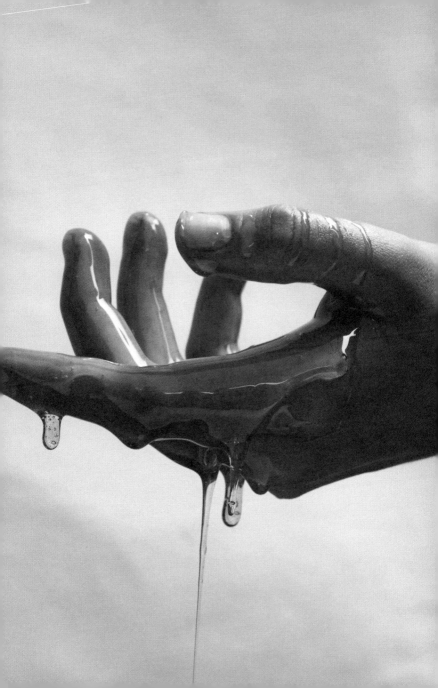

HAND MOISTURISERS & MASKS

Winter warming hand oil
For all skin types

Dry midwinter hands will revel in this heavenly scented oil. Smother them in it, leave for 15 minutes and pat off the excess. Or slip your oily hands into cotton gloves and sleep on it.

1½ tablespoons olive oil
1 tablespoon avocado oil
5 drops patchouli essential oil
5 drops rose essential oil
2 drops benzoin essential oil

– Combine the oils thoroughly and store in a bottle.

Softening honey clay hand mask
For all skin types

1½ tablespoons white clay
1 tablespoon natural yoghurt
2 teaspoons honey

– Combine the ingredients thoroughly.
– Spread over the hands, leave for 10–20 minutes, then rinse off.

Non-greasy lavender & rosemary hand cream
For all skin types

This is the hand cream to have with you at all times.

OIL PHASE
8 g (¼ oz) plant-derived emulsifying wax
2 g (¹⁄₁₆ oz) cocoa butter
2 teaspoons sweet almond oil
2 drops rosemary leaf extract

– Follow the instructions for making an emulsion on page 38.

Honey hand-steaming mask
For all skin types

When your hands are looking a little worn or lacklustre, slather them in honey then steam them for 5–10 minutes over a bowl of hot water containing emollient and healing herbs, like licorice root, chamomile, elderflower, calendula and marshmallow root. Rinse with oatmeal in water and then apply a moisturiser. Slip on a pair of cotton gloves and sleep on it.

Brightening hand mask
For mature skin with uneven pigmentation

Liver spots appear with age and as a result of accumulated exposure to the sun. They respond well to regular exfoliation and foods rich in AHAs and vitamin C. Bicarbonate of soda has a skin brightening effect. Shield the hands from the sun with an SPF sunscreen to prevent further pigmentation.

2 teaspoons lemon juice
2 teaspoons bicarbonate of soda (baking soda)
2 teaspoons powdered buttermilk

– Combine the ingredients thoroughly.
– Spread over the hands, leave for 20–30 minutes, then rinse off. Apply twice a week until your notice a difference. Follow with a protective hand cream.

NAILS & CUTICLES

The condition of the nails and cuticles depends on a healthy diet rich in vitamins and minerals. Harsh chemicals, chlorine from swimming pools and overuse of nail enamel, as well as other aggressive external factors, can wreak havoc on your nails, causing brittleness, splitting and ragged cuticles, hangnails and infection. I find that the contents of a vitamin E capsule or a touch of wheat germ oil massaged into the nails and cuticles daily is a wonderfully simple preventative treatment.

Nail soaks
For weak or brittle nails

To strengthen nails, soak them in a herbal infusion of horsetail for 5 minutes daily. The stems of the horsetail plant are rich in silica, which is vital for healthy nails, bones and hair. Apple cider vinegar is also effective; soak your fingertips in a shallow bowl for 5 minutes. Buttermilk is a wonderful cleanser, nourisher and softener; soak your nails in it, then push back the cuticles with a wooden cuticle stick covered in cotton makeup pads.

Nail-strengthening oil
For weak or brittle nails

Most topical nail strengtheners found on the shelves work by drying out the nails' vital oils, making them brittle. Soaking your nails in a good vegetable oil is a much healthier option. This mixture can be massaged into nails morning and night to keep them flexible and strong, and prevent brittleness, hangnails and ragged cuticles. It will also stimulate circulation, therefore encouraging better growth.

    2 tablespoons sweet almond oil
    2 teaspoons vitamin E oil
    15 drops lemon essential oil
    10 drops frankincense essential oil

– Combine the oils thoroughly.
– Massage into the skin at the base of the nail and over the nail itself.

Nail-fix oil

For minor nail infections

> 2 tablespoons wheat germ oil
> 10 drops tea-tree essential oil
> 10 drops lavender essential oil

– Thoroughly combine the oils and store in a small bottle.
– Rub a few drops into the infected area 3 times a day until the infection clears.

Garden grit trick!

To get rid of ingrained dirt under the fingernails, dig them into lemon halves then scrub vigorously with apple cider vinegar.

NAIL POLISHES

Toluene and formaldehyde, used widely in commercial cosmetic polishes, can cause throat irritation, rashes, headache, nausea and asthma. But if you are partial to a little polish, there are a few good natural alternatives.

Try buffing your nails with beeswax, cocoa butter or a tiny amount of vegetable oil and a soft cloth. Naturally buffed and nicely shaped nails look luxuriously pampered. Buffing is good for your nails, as it stimulates circulation in the nail bed, helping the nails get stronger. Be sure to buff them in an up-and-down motion, as this stimulates blood flow and creates a glorious sheen.

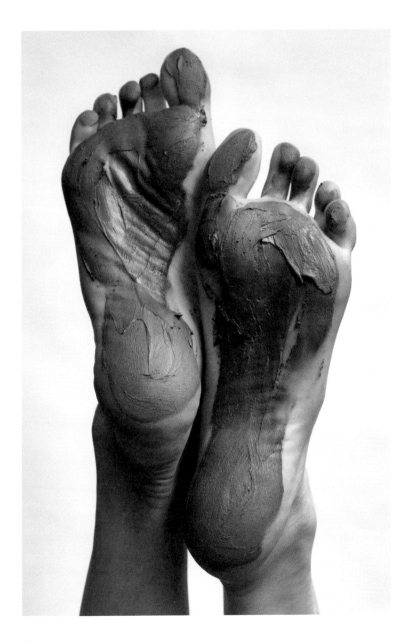

Feet

There's no question that our feet do much of the heavy lifting in our lives – and tired tootsies can certainly make for a tired face. In many ancient cultures, there is a belief that feet must be in contact with the natural elements, so, make a practice out of 'grounding' yourself as much as possible. Walk in the dewy grass, splash in the ocean, or opt for barefoot strolls during summer. Shoes also trap energy around the feet and over a period of time, can make you feel more fatigued. This is one reason why shoes are never worn in Indian temples.

Having good posture, soaking your feet in a soothing footbath and massaging them with an aromatherapy oil will make a huge impact on how you feel. And your feet will also thank you.

REFLEXOLOGY

The ancient healing art of reflexology is based on the belief that every organ of the body is connected to reflex points in the foot, hand or ear. By massaging the feet for 10 minutes each day you are helping to release any blockages in the body and to bring it into balance.

Start out by kneading the soles firmly. The big toe is said to represent the head; gently pull each big toe and carefully rotate it – this will help relieve a stiff neck and tense shoulders. Use both hands to wring out your foot like a damp cloth and tap it to stimulate circulation. Squeeze the area above the heel, around the ankle, which is said to represent the reproductive organs, and press down firmly on any sore points.

Aromatherapy foot oil

20 drops essential oils
5 tablespoons sweet almond oil

– Add the essential oils to the almond oil and mix thoroughly. Store in an airtight bottle.

Some suggested essential oil combinations are:

warming – 14 drops grapefruit, 3 ginger, 3 clove

cooling and energising – 10 drops mandarin, 6 lemongrass, 4 peppermint

relaxing – 8 drops lavender, 8 orange, 4 ylang-ylang

fungal infections – 20 drops palmarosa, 20 thyme, 10 myrrh.

Revitalising foot & leg massage oil

An infused oil of rosemary and lavender (page 33) makes an excellent massage oil for the feet and legs.

FOOT SCRUBS & MASKS

Any ground grain or flour works well on the hard parts of the foot when mixed with a cold-pressed vegetable oil. Salt and sugar scrubs are wonderfully invigorating and slough off tough bits superbly. On hot summer days at the beach, use the rough granules of sand and softening sea water to exfoliate your feet. The simplest way to remove dead skin from the feet and prevent the skin from cracking is to scrub them regularly with a pumice stone. Follow with a refreshing foot scrub.

Overnight heel-softening treatment

To remove a build-up of hard, dead skin, soak feet for 15 minutes in a warm to hot footbath containing 2 tablespoons of bicarbonate of soda (baking soda). Pat feet dry, then rub over a mixture of ¼ cup of olive oil and 2 tablespoons of apple cider vinegar. Pop on your socks and sleep on it.

Lemon-half heel scrub

For all skin types

To soften rough elbows and heels, fill empty lemon halves with sugar, place your elbows or heels in them and rub firmly.

Salt & seaweed scrub

This is a delicious antibacterial, softening and detoxifying foot scrub. You can vary the essential oils as follows: *skin-strengthening and circulation-improving* – geranium; *antiseptic, antifungal and uplifting* – lemon. The kelp will help soften and smooth the skin.

    210 g (7½ oz/1 cup) medium-textured sea salt
    2 tablespoons green clay
    1 teaspoon powdered kelp (optional)
    30 drops lemon or lemon myrtle essential oil

– Combine the ingredients together well and store in an airtight container.
– Combine 2 tablespoons of the mix to form a gritty paste. Massage into the feet using circular motions, paying particular attention to areas with built-up hard skin.

Warming coconut & spice foot paste

Massage this smoothing, softening, uplifting and sensual paste all over the feet and body. Essential oils of jasmine, rose, patchouli and ylang-ylang can be added for an exquisite aroma.

    1½ tablespoons coconut milk
    2 tablespoons oatmeal
    2 teaspoons sweet almond oil
    1 teaspoon mixed spice

– Combine the ingredients to form a smooth paste.
– Massage over the feet, leave for up to 20 minutes, then rinse off.

FOOTBATHS

A good old-fashioned foot soak makes a wonderful alternative to a body bath. Soaking your feet for 10–15 minutes relaxes and revives and has countless therapeutic properties. It helps reduce swelling, prevents varicose veins, treats cellulite and quells any fire in the mind. Herbs, oils and salts make wonderful therapeutic additions to footbaths.

COLD Stand in cold water up to your calves for 2 minutes in the morning. This will invigorate your body and mind in preparation for the day.

LEMON A footbath of 125 ml (4 fl oz) lemon juice (or vinegar) in a basin of water will revive the feet, relieve itchiness and treat athlete's foot.

PEBBLES For a tactile, sensuous soak, rub your feet slowly and firmly over a dozen or so small stones placed at the bottom of your favourite footbath.

Honey & ginger footbath

Ginger promotes circulation and is very warming for winter. Add
2 teaspoons of ground ginger and 2 tablespoons of honey to a bowl
of hot water. This is also an excellent remedy for a thick, unrelenting
head cold, or for warding off a chill.

Herbal deodorising footbath

The warmth and sweat generated by the feet provide the perfect
environment for bacteria to grow, often leading to smelly feet.
Thankfully, they can be treated with good foot hygiene and the frequent
use of deodorising footbaths and foot powders. This wonderfully
soothing and invigorating bath will freshen even the most tainted
tootsies. Other effective deodorising herbs are basil, bay leaves,
eucalyptus, lemon balm, lemongrass, lovage, marjoram, parsley,
spearmint and thyme. Black tea laced with lemon juice also works
wonders, and lemon and orange peel make wonderful healing and
fragrant additions.

    2 tablespoons dried lemon zest
    3 teaspoons dried lavender
    2 teaspoons dried peppermint leaves
    2 teaspoons dried rosemary leaves
    2 teaspoons dried sage leaves

– Add all the ingredients to a half-filled hot footbath and let the herbs infuse
  for 20 minutes.
– Fill the bath with hot water and soak your feet for 10 minutes.

Deodorising forest footbath

This combination will help diminish perspiration and leave the feet smelling like they have just frolicked through an evergreen forest.

8 drops rosemary essential oil
6 drops cypress essential oil
6 drops pine essential oil
2 tablespoons vodka
1 tablespoon cold-pressed vegetable oil

– Drop the essential oils into the vodka and stir well.
– Pour the mixture into a basin of hot water.
– Add the vegetable oil and swish around.
– Adjust the temperature with hot or cold water and soak your feet.

Soothing bath salts

Lavender is a natural pain reliever with relaxing and analgesic properties, while geranium and orange reduce swelling and help the body unwind. The clay will impart enhanced healing properties.

250 g (7½ oz/1¼ cups) Epsom salts
2 teaspoons green clay (optional)
20 drops orange essential oil
10 drops geranium essential oil
10 drops lavender essential oil

– Combine the dry ingredients.
– Add the essential oils drop by drop, stirring until well mixed.
– Transfer to an airtight jar and leave for a week before using.
– Add 2 tablespoons to a basin of warm water.

Body

FOOT POWDERS

Homemade foot powders are a superb alternative to talcum powder, which in recent years has been linked to a number of chronic health conditions. Cornflour (cornstarch), potato flour, arrowroot flour, rice flour, orris root flour and white clay are all ideal, used individually or together. They absorb moisture and perspiration and can be brushed alone over the feet to ease blisters and help remedy fungal infections like athlete's foot (especially bicarbonate of soda). Dried herbs and essential oils make fabulous additions. The following powders will last up to 1 year in the fridge.

Fresh foot powder

40 g (1¼ oz/⅓ cup) cornflour (cornstarch) or orris root powder
70 g (2½ oz/⅓ cup) bicarbonate of soda (baking soda)
50 g (1¾ oz/⅓ cup) white Argiletz clay (or kaolin)
2 tablespoons herbs and flowers, dried and ground (optional)
20 drops essential oils

- Combine the flour and bicarbonate of soda with the clay and herbs (if using).
- Add the essential oils drop by drop, stirring constantly.
- Sift then store in a tightly lidded container with holes punched in the top, or in a salt or parmesan shaker. Shake well before each use.

Here are some essential oil suggestions:

FOR FUNGAL INFECTIONS – 8 drops lavender, 8 tea-tree, 4 lemon

REFRESHING AND DEODORISING – 8 drops cypress, 6 bergamot, 6 grapefruit

EARTHING AND HEALING – 8 drops orange, 6 geranium, 6 patchouli

INVIGORATING – 10 drops lavender, 6 rosemary, 4 spearmint

FOOT MOISTURISERS

Cool & calm foot cream

Keep your feet smooth with this cooling, soothing and easily absorbed moisturising cream. It will last for up to 1 year in the fridge.

OIL PHASE

7 g (¼ oz) plant-derived emulsifying wax

3 g (¹⁄₁₀ oz) cocoa butter

15 ml (½ fl oz) sweet almond oil

5 drops rosemary leaf extract

WATER PHASE

75 ml (2½ fl oz) purified water

5 ml (⅛ fl oz) vegetable glycerine

12 drops grapefruit seed extract

THIRD PHASE

25 drops mandarin essential oil

5 drops peppermint essential oil

– Follow the instructions for making an emulsion on page 38.

Buttery hand & foot treatment balm

This is a rich balm for dry, cracked and damaged hands and feet. Myrrh's healing properties have long been revered. Calendula is also exceptionally effective on rough, callused skin.

OIL PHASE

9 g (¼ oz) plant-derived emulsifying wax

2 g (¹⁄₁₆ oz) shea butter

5 g (⅛ oz) cocoa butter

20 ml (¾ fl oz) calendula-infused oil

6 drops rosemary leaf extract

WATER PHASE

60 ml (2 fl oz) rosewater

5 ml (⅛ fl oz) glycerine

10 drops grapefruit seed extract

THIRD PHASE

15 drops lavender essential oil

5 drops myrrh essential oil

5 drops lemongrass essential oil

– Follow the instructions for making an emulsion on page 38.

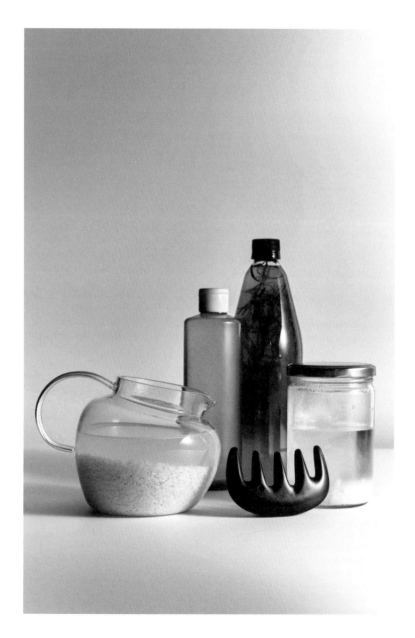

Hair

Your crowning glory or an unruly tangle? The condition of your hair is a good barometer of your state of health and wellbeing (although with the amount of colouring, straightening, curling, blow-drying and styling products we inflict on our tresses, it would be hard to tell!). Your nails, skin, teeth and hair are always last in line when your system distributes nutrients, so you must eat a well-balanced diet if you want lovely hair. Lack of sleep, hormones and sad spirits will also manifest themselves in dull, lifeless hair and sometimes in hair loss.

The first step towards shiny, lustrous hair is to banish harsh shampoos. Like skin, hair is naturally acidic, and regular washing with alkaline shampoos will upset the acid balance and damage your strands. Many people I know have ceased using such shampoos and have found that their dandruff and hair loss have eased.

Your hair will be full of residues from the chemical formulations you have been using, so it will take a little while for natural treatments to remove this build-up, and for your hair to feel soft and look shiny.

HANDY HAIR TIPS

Head & scalp massage

Massaging the hair and scalp stimulates the body's systems, including the glands, nerves and circulation, promoting hair growth and reducing dandruff.

Rice water rinse

Long before the internet, Japanese court ladies would rinse their long, glossy manes with water made from washing rice. Touting benefits including hair strength, shine and growth, it's an easy and inexpensive treatment to try at home. Add 2 cups of uncooked rice to 4 cups of water in a bowl. Cover and leave in a cool, dark area overnight for 8–10 hours. Strain the rice water into a bottle.

The best way to do a rice water treatment is to rinse your hair with it between shampooing and conditioning. Make sure to saturate the strands and scalp and massage the liquid into your roots.

Hair shine protective oil

To protect your hair from chlorine and salt, rinse your hair in fresh water before plunging into a pool or the ocean. Or apply a little of this exquisitely scented oil to protect hair from the sun or sea. Pearl divers wear ylang-ylang oil in their hair for this reason.

2 tablespoons coconut oil (at room temperature)
2 tablespoons jojoba oil
10 drops ylang-ylang essential oil

– Pour or drop the oils into a bottle and shake well to combine.

Hair clean-up

To eliminate shampoo build-up, rinse your hair with 85 g (3 oz/½ cup) of bicarbonate of soda (baking soda) in 250 ml (8½ fl oz/1 cup) of warm water. Rinse well. Soda water also works well as a hair rinse.

Dandruff treatment

Dandruff can be caused by a number of things, such as an inadequate diet, insufficient brushing, shampoo build-up, aggressive hair products and bad scalp circulation. Avoid medicated shampoos; they may relieve dandruff in a day or so, but it will often come back worse than before. Use once a week.

    5 tablespoons jojoba oil
    8 drops lavender essential oil
    6 drops rosemary essential oil
    6 drops tea-tree essential oil

– Mix together and bottle.
– Massage 1–2 tablespoons into damp hair. Leave in hair for 30 minutes.
– Shampoo and condition as normal.

HAIR LOSS

Hair loss may happen gradually or in clumps at various stages of our lives and can be triggered by a number of factors, including hormonal shifts. The good news is it can be helped by using stimulating and nourishing ingredients.

Hair replenishing oil

For all hair types

This is a great oil to stimulate the scalp and keep your hair strong and healthy.

    5 tablespoons jojoba oil
    10 drops atlas cedarwood or clary sage essential oil
    10 drops rosemary essential oil

– Mix together and bottle.
– Massage 1–2 tablespoons into damp hair, and leave on for 30 minutes.
– Shampoo and condition as normal.

HAIR TREATMENT OILS

Jojoba oil lubricates, improves shine and lustre, restores damaged hair, strengthens the hair shaft and treats scalp imbalances. Other vegetable oils are also beneficial, including apricot kernel, castor, coconut, olive and sweet almond oil.

Combine 2½ tablespoons of jojoba oil, coconut oil or another vegetable oil with these essential oil combinations and massage into the hair and scalp. Cover with a plastic shower cap or cling film and a warm, damp towel. Use at least once a week and leave for at least 30 minutes or overnight to allow the oil to penetrate the hair shaft. Rinse, then shampoo.

Also use them in your base shampoos: *normal hair* – 15 drops geranium, 15 lavender; *oily* – 20 drops bergamot, 10 drops patchouli; *dry* – 15 drops sandalwood, 15 drops ylang-ylang; *fragile* – 15 drops carrot seed, 15 drops lavender.

Fragrant hair oil

For all hair types

This sensual blend of oils will keep your hair lustrous and healthy. Your hair makes a great fixative for fragrance.

    20 drops jojoba oil
    10 drops sandalwood essential oil
    5 drops bergamot essential oil
    5 drops clary sage essential oil
    5 drops jasmine essential oil
    5 drops rose essential oil

– Combine the oils thoroughly.
– Place 3 drops on the fingertips and/or on your hairbrush and run through your hair.

SHAMPOOS

Many commercial shampoos contain sodium lauryl sulfate, a skin irritant, so ensure that your shampoo is sulfate-free. Most homemade shampoos do not lather like bought shampoos, but will keep your hair as clean and in excellent condition. Shampoo your hair only when it really needs it, and use lukewarm water for shampooing and cold water for the final rinse.

Quickie shampoos

For all hair types

Buy a mild, pH-balanced, sulfate-free shampoo base at a health food shop and add 20 drops of essential oil for every 5 tablespoons of shampoo.

Deep conditioning Castile shampoo

Eggs have been used to cleanse and condition hair for generations because of their cleansing and moisturising properties. This is a fabulous simple, fragrant conditioning shampoo for all hair types. I use this recipe often to revive and add lustre to my hair. It also tames flyaways.

½ teaspoon liquid Castile shampoo base
1 egg yolk
2 drops essential oil to suit your hair type (pages 170–1)

– Combine the ingredients thoroughly.

Dry shampoo
For all hair types

Flours absorb impurities from the hair, get rid of that greasy look and are great when you can't shampoo your hair. White clay and orris root powder also work very well.

10 drops essential oils of your choice
40 g (1½ oz/⅓ cup) cornflour (cornstarch)

– Add the essential oils to the cornflour drop by drop, mixing thoroughly to avoid clumps.
– Sift.
– Massage small quantities into your hair, close to your scalp. Use a brush to distribute the mixture and to begin to remove it, then tip your head upside down and continue brushing to remove the rest.

Zesty orange clay shampoo
For oily hair

This cleansing and balancing shampoo will also help whisk dead skin away from the scalp.

5 tablespoons shampoo base
2 teaspoons green clay
10 drops orange essential oil
10 drops ylang-ylang essential oil

– Combine the ingredients thoroughly.

CONDITIONERS

Conditioners are especially useful if your hair has been over-coloured or otherwise chemically treated. When your body is healthy and balanced and you are using gentle, natural shampoos, you may find that you don't even need to condition. Leave conditioners on for at least 5 minutes after shampooing, then rinse out.

Quickie conditioner
For all hair types

Add 20 drops of essential oils to suit your hair type (pages 170–1) to 5 tablespoons of a herbal conditioner base from a health food shop.

CONDITIONING TREATMENTS & MASKS

Hot oil & ginger hair rehab
For damaged hair

Natural oils have been used as conditioners to nourish the hair for centuries. This simple recipe restores damaged hair and eradicates dandruff. Warming the oil before use helps it better penetrate the hair shaft.

> 3 tablespoons cold-pressed olive oil
> 2 teaspoons ginger root juice

- Heat the olive oil in a bain-marie, stirring until warm.
- Remove from the heat, add the ginger root juice and whisk rapidly.
- Massage through the hair and scalp then cover with a wet, hot towel for 1 hour. Rinse in warm water. Finish with a cold rinse and shampoo and condition as normal.

Egg masks

For oily or dry hair

Egg masks are highly nutritive and can help give your mane a lovely lustre and shine. For oily hair mix 2 egg whites with 1 tablespoon brewer's yeast. For dry hair, mix 2 egg yolks with 1 tablespoon olive oil.

Frizz-fix avocado hair mask

For dry hair

Sleeping on the finest silk pillow slips and patting your freshly washed and dried tresses with a few drops of jojoba oil will help tame frizziness, as will this great mask.

2 tablespoons natural yoghurt
1 tablespoon olive oil
½ avocado

– Mash the avocado into the combined oil and yoghurt to form a creamy paste. To smooth out any lumps, you can use a blender.
– Apply to damp hair, leave for 30 minutes, then rinse thoroughly.
– Shampoo and condition as normal.

RINSES

Rinses can be made from vinegars, or herbal vinegars, infusions and decoctions. They are effective in balancing and healing both the scalp and the hair. A cool rinse can also help close the hair cuticles, resulting in greater shine.

Parsley & peppermint rinse

For all hair types

A strong infusion of parsley will help heal the scalp while stimulating the hair and helping to balance the sebaceous glands. It also helps control flyaways. If your hair is very greasy, add 1 tablespoon of lemon juice.

125 ml (4 fl oz/½ cup) peppermint infusion
125 ml (4 fl oz/½ cup) parsley infusion

– Combine the infusions.
– After shampooing, massage into the scalp and hair. Follow with conditioner as normal.

Vinegar rinses
For all hair types

Apple cider vinegar makes an excellent rinse, especially if you suffer from a flaky dry scalp. It helps re-establish the acid pH of your scalp and minimise the build-up of hair products and debris. It also helps close the cuticles along the hair shaft, leaving hair smooth and manageable and helping with flyaways. Don't worry, the strong fermented scent of the vinegar will not stay in your hair if rinsed well and followed by conditioner.

Add 1 tablespoon of apple cider vinegar to a glass of tepid water, pour it over your hair after shampooing and massage into the scalp before rinsing. Alternatively, add 1 tablespoon of a herbal vinegar to 250 ml (8½ fl oz/1 cup) of water, massage into your scalp and pour through your hair. Finish with a rinse of cold water or herbal infusion. Burdock root, chamomile, dried nettle, horsetail, lavender, peppermint, rosemary, sage and thyme are all stimulating and restorative herbs for the hair and scalp. Use herbs to suit your hair type (pages 170–1).

HAIR-STYLING AIDS

Hair sprays often contain plastics and other synthetic chemicals that you probably shouldn't breathe in or apply to your hair and scalp. Fortunately, there are some impressive homemade alternatives that work wonders.

Detangling spray

For all hair types

Rosemary oil is a blessing when your hair is an unruly tangle. It is essential to shake the bottle before each use, to disperse the rosemary oil throughout the mix.

4 drops rosemary essential oil (or chamomile for blonde hair)

10 drops lavender essential oil

5 tablespoons aloe vera juice

1 teaspoon vegetable glycerine

– Add all the ingredients together in a bottle.

– This will last up to 3 months in the fridge. Shake before use.

Lime & coconut hair wax

For all hair types

This fabulous hair balm will help control and add shine to short hair. Coconut oil is renowned for its restorative properties and has been used for centuries as a skin and hair polish.

15 g beeswax

3 tablespoons coconut oil

2 tablespoons olive oil

20 drops lime essential oil

– Melt the beeswax and cocoa butter in a bain-marie, mixing well to combine.

– Remove from heat for a few minutes, then add the essential oils.

– Pour into a small jar then allow to solidify at room temperature. Store in the fridge.

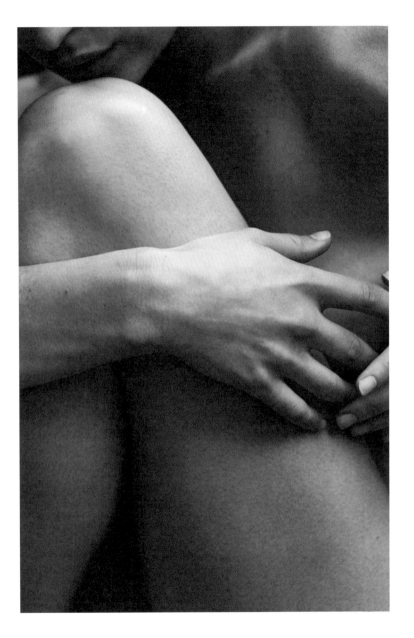

Sun care
& sunburn

The sun used sensibly is a wonderful beauty aid. It releases
feel-good hormones into your system and provides the body with
vitamin D, which is essential for bone, gut, skin and immune health.
But, like everything, the sun is best in moderation and skin should
always be protected with a minimum of SPF30.

A diet rich in antioxidants, including vibrantly coloured fruits and
vegetables, green tea and cocoa will also help to protect your skin
from free radicals that are generated by sun exposure – as will using
nourishing, antioxidant rich skincare. Many plant oils, such as sesame
or raspberry seed boast a natural SPF, but their protection is minimal,
so while they may help as part of a holistic approach to suncare, they
are not a replacement for an effective SPF product.

Plants are clever; they contain compounds that can assist to repair,
relieve, replenish and rejuvenate inflamed and sun-damaged skin.
Rich in nutrients and essential fatty acids, they make wonderful
after-sun beauty aids.

AFTER-SUN BEAUTY AIDS

Avoiding sunburn is important to keep your skin and body healthy, however if you do happen to get sunburnt, slather these relieving and healing ingredients onto your skin.

ALOE VERA GEL fresh from the leaf or bought at a health food shop.

APPLE CIDER VINEGAR diluted in water.

BLACK TEA contains tannic acid that will help remove the heat from sunburn. Apply cool.

MILK, BUTTERMILK AND YOGHURT are all soothing.

OATS are very soothing. Wrap in muslin (cheesecloth), soak in warm water and rub over sun-kissed areas.

TOMATOES, POTATOES, CUCUMBERS OR APPLES Mash or grate the flesh or use the juice.

WITCH HAZEL, COOL NETTLE, SAGE OR CHAMOMILE TEA Freeze wet tea bags and apply them for further relief.

Sunburn blister relief

Dust cornflour, potato flour or rice flour dusted over blisters.

Sun-kissed skin spray

This is a wonderfully healing and refreshing tonic for the skin, whether sun-parched or not. Store in a spray bottle in the fridge and it will last you the summer. Spray this over the hair for shine and protection, and to prevent frizziness.

10 drops lavender essential oil
1 teaspoon apple cider vinegar
250 ml (8½ fl oz/1 cup) aloe vera juice
contents of 2–3 vitamin E capsules

– Add the essential oil to the vinegar, then mix in the aloe vera and vitamin E.
– Store in a spray bottle and shake well before use. Keep refrigerated.

Sun-down radiance oil

For all skin types

This rejuvenating oil will help to nourish the skin. The scent is both calming and uplifting, perfect for wearing on a summer's night.

125 ml (4 fl oz) unrefined sesame oil
2 tablespoons calendula-infused oil
2 teaspoons vitamin E oil
10 drops lavender essential oil
10 drops mandarin essential oil
5 drops ylang-ylang essential oil

– Combine the oils thoroughly.

Guide to essential oils, herbs, floral waters & foods

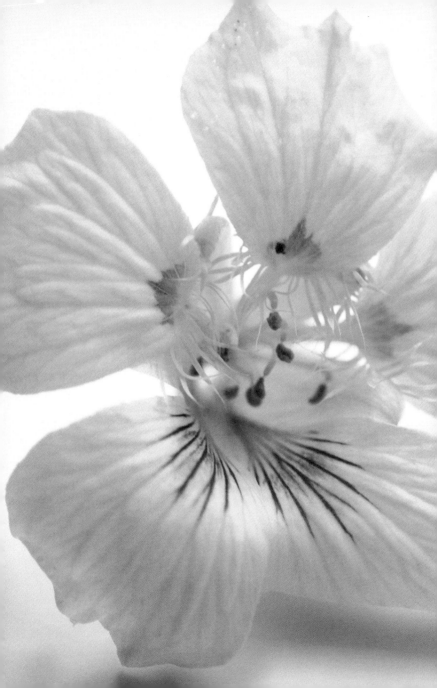

SKIN TYPES OR CONDITIONS

All & normal

ESSENTIAL OILS chamomile, geranium, jasmine, lavender, neroli, patchouli, rose, rosewood, ylang-ylang

HERBS aloe vera, black tea, calendula, chamomile, comfrey, elderflower, gotu kola, green tea, lavender, licorice root, marshmallow, parsley, rosehip, soapwort

FLORAL WATERS chamomile, jasmine, lavender, orange blossom, rose

FOODS almond meal, apple, cucumber, grape, honey, lettuce, melon, oats, papaya (pawpaw), pear, potato, rice, seaweed, wheat germ, yoghurt

MILKS buttermilk, coconut milk goat's milk, kefir, rice milk, soy milk, yoghurt

OILS apricot kernel, grape seed, jojoba, safflower, sunflower, sweet almond

Oily

ESSENTIAL OILS atlas cedarwood, bergamot, cypress, geranium, juniper, lavender, lemon, lime, mandarin, orange, tangerine, ylang-ylang

HERBS alfalfa, aloe vera, bay leaves, burdock root, dandelion, lavender, lemon balm, lemon verbena, raspberry leaves, rosemary, sage, tumeric, witch hazel, yarrow

FLORAL WATERS lavender, witch hazel

FOODS apricots, cabbage, carrot, egg white, grape, grapefruit, honey, lemon, lemon zest, lime, mandarin, orange, papaya (pawpaw), pineapple, strawberry, tomato, watercress, yeast

MILKS buttermilk, full-fat or nut milk, kefir, yoghurt

OILS apricot kernel, hazelnut, jojoba, sweet almond

Dry

ESSENTIAL OILS jasmine, lavender, palmarosa, patchouli, rose, sandalwood

HERBS aloe vera, calendula, chamomile, comfrey root, elderflower, licorice root, marshmallow root, parsley

FLORAL WATERS jasmine, rose

FOODS avocado, banana, carrot, egg yolk, honey, lecithin, melon, papaya (pawpaw), pear, tahini

MILKS cream, full-fat milk, goat's milk, kefir, soy milk, yoghurt

OILS avocado, borage seed, macadamia nut, olive, wheat germ

Combination

ESSENTIAL OILS geranium, lavender, neroli, palmarosa, sandalwood, ylang-ylang

HERBS see 'all' and 'oily'

FLORAL WATERS lavender, orange blossom

FOODS see 'all' and 'oily'

MILKS see 'all' and 'oily'

OILS apricot kernel, jojoba, sesame, sweet almond

Sensitive

ESSENTIAL OILS everlasting, German chamomile, jasmine, lavender, neroli, rose, rosewood, sandalwood, yarrow

HERBS aloe vera, ashgwhandha, calendula, chamomile, comfrey, gotu kola, green tea, licorice, marshmallow, red clover, soapwort

FLORAL WATERS chamomile, orange blossom, rose

FOODS apple, avocado, banana, honey, melon, oatmeal, papaya (pawpaw), pear, wheat germ

MILKS buttermilk, coconut milk, goat's milk, kefir, soy milk, yoghurt

OILS apricot kernel, calendula infused, jojoba, sweet almond

Dehydrated

ESSENTIAL OILS palmarosa, rose, rosewood, sandalwood

HERBS aloe vera, comfrey root, marshmallow root, parsley, rose, slippery elm

FLORAL WATERS chamomile, orange blossom, rose

FOODS apple, cucumber, melon, pear

MILKS coconut milk, full-fat milk, kefir, rice milk, soy milk, yoghurt

OILS apricot kernel, jojoba, sweet almond

Mature

ESSENTIAL OILS carrot seed, everlasting, fennel, frankincense, jasmine, lavender, myrrh, patchouli, rose, rosewood, sandalwood, ylang-ylang

HERBS elderflower, fennel seed, ginseng, gotu kola, green tea, parsley, rose geranium, sage, shiitake mushroom

FLORAL WATERS jasmine, rose

FOODS almond meal, avocado, banana, carrot, egg, honey, orange juice, papaya (pawpaw), peach, tahini, tomato

MILKS coconut milk, cream, full-fat milk, kefir, soy milk, yoghurt

OILS avocado, borage, carrot infused, evening primrose, jojoba, macadamia, olive, rosehip, wheat germ

Acneous

ESSENTIAL OILS bergamot, cedarwood, clary sage, cypress, eucalyptus, everlasting, geranium, chamomile, grapefruit, juniper, lavender, lemon, myrrh, palmarosa, patchouli, petitgrain, pine, Roman chamomile, tea tree, thyme, yarrow

HERBS aloe vera, burdock root, calendula, chamomile, comfrey, dandelion, echinacea, eucalyptus, garlic, gotu kola, lemon balm, lemongrass, nasturtium flowers, sage, thyme, yarrow

FLORAL WATERS lavender, witch hazel

FOODS alfalfa, apricot, cabbage, carrot, grapefruit, lemon juice and zest, lime juice and zest, Manuka honey, plum, strawberry, tomato, turmeric, watercress, yeast

MILKS coconut milk, kefir, rice milk, full-fat or nut milk, yoghurt

OILS borage, castor, evening primrose, hazelnut, jojoba

Devitalised

ESSENTIAL OILS grapefruit, lemongrass, peppermint, rosemary, vetiver

HERBS coriander, fennel seed, horsetail, lemongrass, lemon verbena, nettle, parsley, rosemary

FLORAL WATERS orange blossom, witch hazel

FOODS bicarbonate of soda (baking soda), citrus fruit, lemon juice, papaya (pawpaw), strawberry, tomato, yeast

Dermatitis/Eczema

ESSENTIAL OILS benzoin, everlasting, German chamomile, lavender, myrrh, palmarosa, patchouli, sandalwood, yarrow, ylang-ylang

HERBS aloe vera, ashwagandha, burdock root, calendula, chamomile, chickweed, comfrey, dandelion leaf and root, licorice root, marshmallow root, red clover, yarrow

FLORAL WATERS chamomile, rose

FOODS cucumber, green beans, papaya (pawpaw), rockmelon (cantaloupe)

OILS apricot kernel, borage, evening primrose, jojoba, rosehip

Broken capillaries

ESSENTIAL OILS blue chamomile, cypress, geranium, lemon, rose

HERBS gotu kola, parsley

FLORAL WATER rose

OIL carrot seed infused

Body odour

ESSENTIAL OILS atlas cedarwood, bergamot, clary sage, cypress, eucalyptus, frankincense, geranium, lavender, may chang, melissa, myrrh, patchouli, pine, rosewood, sandalwood, tea-tree, ylang-ylang

HERBS geranium, lavender, lemon balm, lemongrass, lovage, peppermint, rosemary, sage, thyme

Scarring

ESSENTIAL OILS benzoin, cypress, frankincense, German chamomile, lavender, myrrh, patchouli, rosewood, sandalwood

HERBS aloe vera, calendula, comfrey, gotu kola

OILS borage, evening primrose, rosehip, vitamin E

Warts

ESSENTIAL OILS lemon, tea tree, thyme

HAIR TYPES OR CONDITIONS

All

ESSENTIAL OILS geranium, lavender, rosemary, ylang-ylang
HERBS chamomile, henna, horsetail, lavender, rosemary, sage

Oily

ESSENTIAL OILS bergamot, cedarwood, cypress, geranium, grapefruit, juniper, lemon, lime, patchouli, petitgrain, rosemary, sage, thyme
HERBS burdock root, lime flowers, nettle, peppermint, thyme, witch hazel, yarrow

Dry & damaged

ESSENTIAL OILS frankincense, geranium, lavender, rosewood, sandalwood

HERBS aloe vera, chamomile, comfrey, marshmallow root, soapwort

Dandruff

ESSENTIAL OILS atlas cedarwood, cajeput, clary sage, eucalyptus, rosemary, spike lavender, tea tree, thyme

HERBS horsetail, lavender, nettle, parsley, peppermint, rosemary, sage, thyme

Inflamed & irritated scalp (with eczema & psoriasis)

ESSENTIAL OILS calendula, German chamomile, lavender, patchouli, sandalwood

HERBS calendula, chamomile, comfrey, lavender, licorice, marshmallow, parsley, soapwort

Hair loss

ESSENTIAL OILS atlas cedarwood, clary sage, ginger, lavender, peppermint, rosemary, thyme, ylang-ylang

HERBS bay, ginger, horsetail, nettle, peppermint, rosemary, thyme

Further reading

Battaglia, Salvatore, *The Complete Guide to Aromatherapy*, International Centre of Holistic Aromatherapy, Brisbane, 2003

Fairley, Josephine, *Organic Beauty*, Dorling Kindersley, Melbourne, 2001

Farrow, Kevin, Skin Deep: *A Guide to Safe, Chemical-free Skincare and Cleaning Products*, Lothian, Melbourne, 2002

Mathews, Megan & Alison Casser, *Radiant Skin, Radiant Health*, ABC Books, Sydney, 2004

Neal's Yard Remedies and Susan Curtis, *Make Your Own Cosmetics*, Aurum Press, London, 1997

Purchon, Nerys, *Bodycraft: Health and Beauty the Natural Way*, Hodder & Stoughton, Sydney, 1993

Rose, Jeanne, *Herbal Body Book*, Grosset & Dunlap, New York, 1976

Stubbin, Carolyn, *Do It Yourself Pure Plant Skin Care*, International Centre of Holistic Aromatherapy, Brisbane, 1999

Tisserand, Robert, *The Art of Aromatherapy*, Daniel, London, 1977

Wildwood, Christine, *Aromatherapy*, Bloomsbury, London, 1996

Worwood, Valerie Ann, *The Fragrant Pharmacy: A Home and Health Care Guide to Aromatherapy and Essential Oils*, Macmillan, London, 1990

Wright, Janet, *Ayurvedic Beauty*, Lorenz Books, London, 2002

Suppliers

NEW DIRECTIONS AUSTRALIA
47 Carrington Road
Marrickville, Sydney
NSW 2204 Australia
phone +61 2 8577 5999

NEAL'S YARD REMEDIES
www.nealsyardremedies.com

Index

Published in 2024 by Hardie Grant Books,
an imprint of Hardie Grant Publishing

Hardie Grant Books (Melbourne)
Wurundjeri Country
Building 1, 658 Church Street
Richmond, Victoria 3121

Hardie Grant North America
2912 Telegraph Ave
Berkeley, California 94705

hardiegrant.com/books

Hardie Grant acknowledges the Traditional
Owners of the Country on which we work,
the Wurundjeri People of the Kulin Nation and
the Gadigal People of the Eora Nation, and
recognises their continuing connection to the
land, waters and culture. We pay our respects
to their Elders past and present.

A catalogue record for this
book is available from the
NATIONAL
LIBRARY   National Library of Australia
OF AUSTRALIA

A catalogue of this book is available from
the National Library of Australia

Feeding Your Skin
ISBN 978 1 76145 062 4
ISBN 978 1 76145 063 1 (ebook)

10 9 8 7 6 5 4 3 2 1

Publisher: Simon Davis
Head of Editorial: Jasmin Chua
Design Manager: Kristin Thomas
Designer: Daniel New
Art Director: Julie Austin
Photographer: Mason Stevenson
Stylist: Caitlin Melling
Model: India Stibilj
Head of Production: Todd Rechner
Production Controller: Jessica Harvie

Colour reproduction by
Splitting Image Colour Studio
Printed in China by Leo Paper Products LTD.

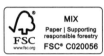

MIX
Paper | Supporting
responsible forestry
FSC   FSC® C020056
www.fsc.org

The paper this book is printed on is from
FSC®-certified forests and other sources.
FSC® promotes environmentally responsible,
socially beneficial and economically viable
management of the world's forests.

Acknowledgements
Thank you to Davor, Kristen, Ash, Sam, Jules,
Caitlin, Mason, India, Lisa, Rosie, Lois, Daniel,
and Roxy, Jasmin and Simon at Hardie Grant.

Disclaimer
The recipes and advice in this book are
intended as a guide only. If you have any skin
issues, infections or other, please check with
a health practitioner. The publisher, its
employees and the author are not liable for
any harm or injury to any person as a result
of the following advice contained in this book;
responsibility for personal health and safety
remains with the reader.

Measurements
Please note that Australian measurements are
used in this book: a standard cup is 250 ml
(8½ fl oz) and a tablespoon is 20 ml (¾ fl oz).